THEY'RE FAKE AND THEY'RE SPECTACULAR!

A Survivor's Guide to Breast Cancer and Beyond

Judy San Roman

The information contained in this book is based upon research both personal and professional experience by the author.It is not intended as a substitute for consulting with your physician or healthcare provider. Any attempt to diagnose and treat illness should be done under the direction of a healthcare professional.

The publisher does not advocate the use of any particular healthcare protocol but believes the information in this book should be available to the public. The publisher and author are not responsible for any adverse effects or consequences resulting from the use of any suggestions, implications or any other preparations or procedures discussed in this book. Should the reader have any questions concerning the appropriateness of any procedures or preparation mentioned, the author and publisher strongly suggest consulting a professional healthcare advisor.

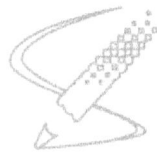

Creative Image Publishing
290 Broadhollow Road,
Melville, NY 11747
Creative Image, www.creativeimage.com

I dedicate this book to my mother, Adriana, you are my guardian angel always.

And to my grandmother, Olga, who lived a long and wonderful life to age 89. She inspired me to be the best person I can be.

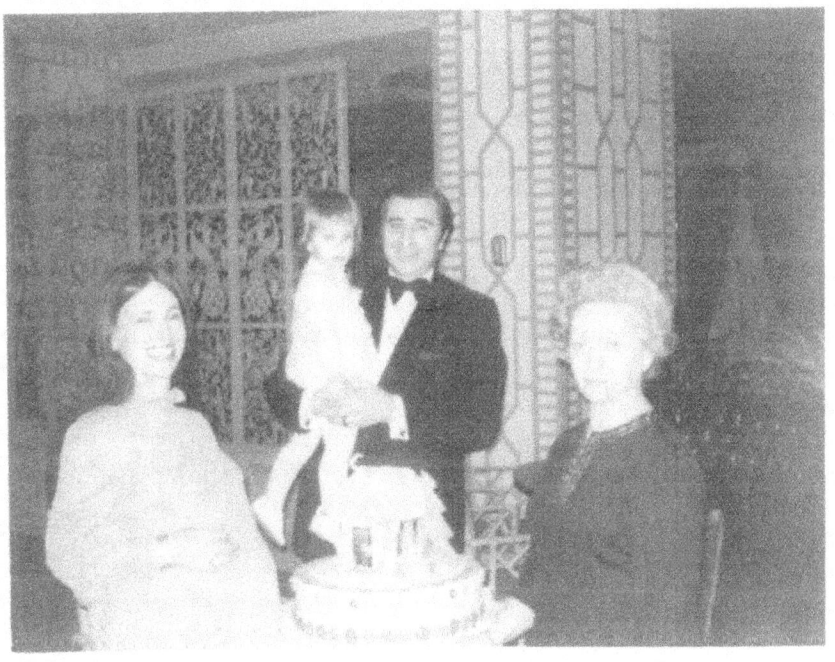

My parents with my grandmother. My brother is in my Mom's belly.

To my Aunt Martha, who beat cancer as well; I love you dearly.

To my best friends, whose love and support I will always cherish. You are and continue to be my prescription for Prozac.

To my network of angels: my doctors, nurses, PAs and staff members who helped me make tough decisions and led me to a speedy recovery.

Dr. Michael Osborne; Thank you for saving my life.

To Greta: Thank you for all your love and showing me courage to beat this. You are my inspiration and hero!

To Tara: You are a wonderful, strong and courageous woman. I love you dearly.

Paulie, God Bless your mother Mary and sister Eileen. They are in our hearts forever.

For all the women who weren't as fortunate as I to beat their cancer, God Bless.

I pray that we can find a cure so that my beautiful niece Jacqueline's generation does not have to endure this terrible disease.

ACKNOWLEDGEMENTS

It is with great pleasure that I acknowledge the contributions of a number of people whose input has been invaluable to this book. First, Dr Ridwan Shabsigh, who had keen insights and passion to push me to write my story and share it with women dealing with cancer. Thank you for assuming my competence before I'd really proven myself.

I would like to thank the expert in the literary world: the passionate and New York Times bestselling author Antonia Felix. You encouraged me and developed my book from my original plan. Thank you for all your hard work, time and love for this manuscript.

Jessica DeBenedetto, you are my heavy and my heart. Thank you for being such an important part of my life.

Leslie, Valerie and Kayla Felix, thank you so much for all the love and support you show me every day of my life. You are AMAZING people!!!! Anne Geiger, for your tough and beautiful love.

To my brother, Josi, thank you for all your love and support.

Rob, Michael, Sachin, James, and Peter D, you are all super brothers. Dr. Gregory La Trenta thank you for your insight, kindness, and support.

Eternal thanks to my girls, Irene, Nazy, Karen, Christy, Dawn, Claudia, Miozoty, Ivette, Kim, Rosanna, Mimi and Sandra. I love you sooooo much!!!

Estrella, eres mi estrella siempre.

Beatriz, mi otra Mama, te quiero mucho.

Mayo/Fragomen family much love and gratitude always.

Daddy, la dolorosa experiencia y sufrimiento que tuvistes con el cancer de mi mama, verlo repitido en tu hija. Dandome siempre fuerzas, besos y amor.

Dr. Carmen Campisi and his lovely wife Cathy your hearts are beautiful.

June, you are a sister to me and a wonderful person. Thank you for all of your love and support always.

Elaine Albert, your strength inspires me.

Dr. Errol Mallett and Denise Wallace much love and champagne always.

Brandon, I love you very much!!!! I still see hearts everywhere because of you.

THEY'RE FAKE AND THEY'RE SPECTACULAR!

Judy San Roman

TABLE OF CONTENTS

Acknowledgements

Preface by Ridwan Shabsigh, M.D.

Foreward by Gregory S. LaTrenta M.D. P.C, F.A.C.S

Chapter 1   THE DIAGNOSIS

Chapter 2   SEARCHING FOR DR. RIGHT

Chapter 3   ON THE TABLE

Chapter 4   CHEMO

Chapter 5   WHEN DEPRESSION IS NOT A DIRTY WORD

Chapter 6   BIG GIRLS DO CRY, AND THEN THEY MOVE ON

Chapter 7   THE NAKED TRUTH

Chapter 8   STAY POSITIVE AND TAKE CONTROL: A FORMULA FOR HOPE

Chapter 9   FRIENDS & FAMILY: BETTER THAN PROZAC

Appendix I: TIPS

Appendix II: RESOURCES

About the Author

PREFACE

Witnessing many patients, as well as some of my friends and relatives, suffer from cancer and other dangerous diseases, I realized that Judy's story could actually help many people deal with their diseases. Looking at the big picture, we in the health care profession can provide an accurate diagnosis and effective treatment, but another factor in the success of health care is the patient. In Judy, I saw a patient taking charge of her life, her disease and its treatments. She dealt with the treatments' side effects and the emotional, psychological and social impact of the disease in a highly effective way. In addition to Judy the patient, I saw in her Judy the human being, who emphasized quality of life in addition to quantity of life. I learned from her how fear turns into determination, depression into hope, despair into courage and bad times into good times.

I contacted Judy and asked to her to write her story and publish it. Although being a urologist puts me far from breast cancer as a medical specialty, I was so convinced that she had something special and life changing to give to others. Once again, Judy impressed me with her courage by agreeing to share with the public all the details of her story, including some very personal issues and experiences. She left nothing out!

Readers should enjoy this real-life story of a woman who wrote her own rulebook for successfully battling cancer.

Ridwan Shabsigh, MD

Brooklyn, October 1, 2008

FOREWORD

The diagnosis of breast cancer for many women means that, along with the shock of discovering that they have breast cancer, they are faced with the need to make some giant and very difficult decisions in an extremely short period of time. For most women this involves obtaining as much information as possible about their disease, their doctors, and the medical centers in which they will choose to have their care. Once these decisions have been made, their thoughts usually drift to the very real possibility that they will lose one or both of their breasts. What to do about replacing their breasts, although perhaps initially thought to be the least important decision for many women, will ultimately work out to be one of their most important. Although afflicting nearly 15 percent of women today, the vast majority of women survive breast cancer, and in a years time, how they look and feel about themselves, their sense of femininity, their sexuality and their sense of well being, will all be deeply interwoven into the reconstructive efforts that are used to recreate their breasts.

When I first met Judy San Roman in March of 2005, she was a beautiful, single 34-year-old executive who had a very strong family history of breast cancer, who already had had multiple breast biopsies performed since she'd been 26, and who recently had been diagnosed with left breast cancer. Although I am certain she was frightened and anxious inside, she radiated warmth, kindness and a true charm on the outside — attributes I knew needed to be nurtured. Although she didn't truly understand it at that time, I knew then that the future held for her a tough year of bilateral mastectomies and reconstruction, chemotherapy and then rebuilding the very fabric of her young life. Her decision to have a bilateral mastectomy and bilateral breast reconstruction with implants meant she would need to devote a 6- to 12-month period of several well-timed operations to build her breasts back. This meant she would need to be committed to her original decision. This decision was reinforced by her recent diagnosis as having the BRAC gene. This gene means that if and when she developed breast cancer, it would likely be persistent and aggressive, develop at a young age, and she would need to chose an extremely aggressive treatment regime. This recent technological advance has quite literally saved lives, as many patients 10-20 years ago did not have this diagnostic test available.

Judy chose to have her care with Dr. Michael Osborne and me in late 2005 and early 2006 at Cornell University Medical Center. Today, she is as warm, vibrant and beautiful a young woman as I could ever have hoped for her to become when I first met her three years ago. The anxiety and fear have been replaced by the zeal of the writer she has become. She radiated that the day I first met her. She has chosen to write this book about her journey, a book well worth reading and celebrating. Had her journey begun in the 1980s when I first began my practice of plastic surgery, the outcome may have been quite different, and this wonderful story may not have been told.

Gregory S. LaTrenta, MD

New York, October 15, 2008

Chapter 1

The Diagnosis

"Without courage you cannot practice any of the other virtues."

—Maya Angelou

All my life I have lived by three golden rules: live well, laugh often and love much. I was the happy kid who always walked around with a smile on her face. More than once my tenth-grade English teacher, Mrs. Cameron, snapped at me for always smiling in class; she must have thought I wasn't paying attention. One of my professors at Queens College in New York noticed it, too, stopping me in the hallway one day to tell me I looked like I was daydreaming about Mr. Wonderful. I didn't tell him what was really on my mind—the sweet, ricotta-filled cannolis I was going to eat in the neighborhood pizzeria after school.

This upbeat attitude was still going strong in February 2005, a couple of days after a routine mammogram. I was 34 years old and filled with the romantic notion about a future with a big family, fulfilling career and lots of friends. As a sales representative for a major pharmaceutical company, I enjoyed a great income and was living the good life. Death wasn't part of the equation until my doctor called and told me to come in to discuss my test results. I had had several scares through the years with cysts that, after being examined through biopsies and ultrasound, turned out to be benign, so every six months I secretly faced the fear of encountering the "m" word—malignant. Doctor Sampath Kumar, my vascular/breast surgeon, had been watching me closely. Like many women I had always had cystic breasts, and that fact, along with my family history of breast cancer, were red flags he would not let me ignore.

I knew that the rule for a woman with a family history of breast cancer is to start getting regular mammograms ten years earlier than the age at which her mother, sister or other relative was diagnosed. I had followed that routine, starting even earlier than necessary at age 25, and so far I'd been lucky.

But when Dr. Kumar called about my latest test, I feared the worst. A picture of my Mom's chest flashed into my mind, an image seared into my memory at age ten when she had undergone a scarring double mastectomy. To my young eyes the healing gashes looked like the mark of Zorro. On TV reruns Zorro was the good guy, leaving his mark after saving the day. But even Zorro couldn't save my Mom.

I let that image go and asked my boyfriend, Michael, to go see Dr. Kumar with me. We took separate cars to the appointment because we planned to go to work afterward. Our relationship was a little shaky at the time, but Michael was very thoughtful and sensitive. He was sad that morning, and I've often thought that maybe we both knew, deep down, what was to come. He had never come to one of my appointments before.

In a few minutes we arrived at the doctor's office in Brooklyn and were asked to wait in an examination room. Dr. Kumar came in and pulled up a stool to sit across from us. There were tears in his eyes as he gently squeezed my upper right arm. "I'm sorry," he said. "We found a growth that is malignant. It's breast cancer, infiltrating ductal

I knew that the rule for a woman with a family history of breast cancer is to start getting regular mammograms ten years earlier than the age at which her mother, sister or other relative was diagnosed. I had followed that routine, starting even earlier than necessary at age 25, and so far I'd been lucky.

15

carcinoma." He paused, and then assured me that because we caught it early we didn't have to think terminal. The tumor was small, less than one centimeter, and it was a very common type of cancer with an excellent cure rate. The news didn't register and I went into automatic pilot. "Good to see you," I said, standing up. "I'll see you in six months." Michael directed me back into my chair. Then reality set in and I saw myself shrinking into a skeleton like my Mom, shuffling back and forth to treatments, recovering slowly and painfully from surgery, trading in my breasts for a torso stretched white with scars, and dying.

The future was blank. I felt empty, shattered. Doctor Kumar had more to say, but I don't remember any of it. We left and drove back to my apartment in our cars, Michael crying on the phone to his best friend, Mike, the entire time. I gripped the steering wheel and tried to figure out what hurt more, imagining how Mom must have felt when she left two kids motherless or picturing myself dying before I had a chance to have kids of my own. For the next twenty minutes I drove the streets while the movie of my childhood played through my mind.

I lived my Mom's battle with cancer first hand. In my first years of grade school, after school meant jumping in an ambulance with her to go to the hospital for chemotherapy and radiation treatments. To the doctors

All About the Breast

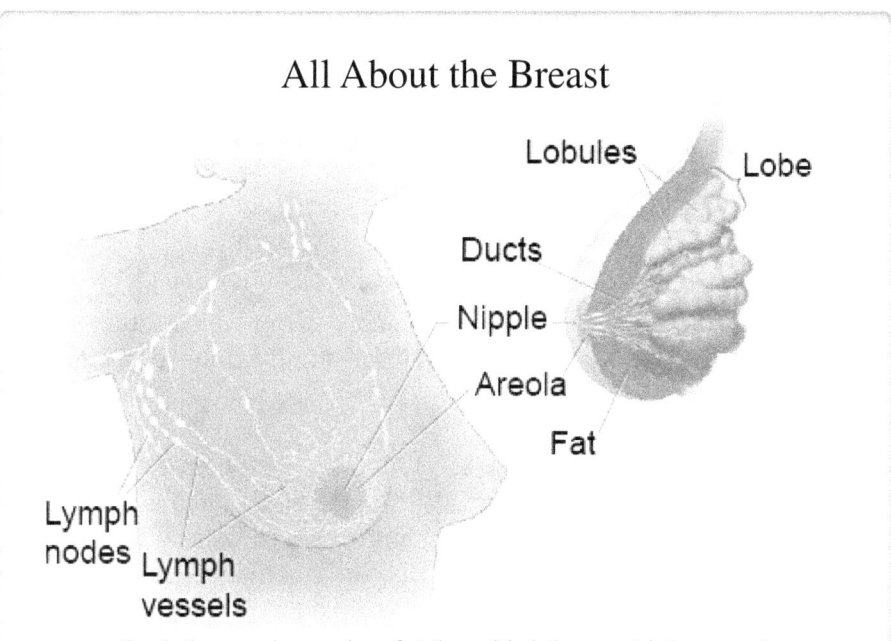

Each breast is made of 15 to 20 lobes, which contain many smaller lobules that carry tiny milk producing glands. Milk flows from the lobules through the thin ducts of the nipple.

The breasts also contain lymph vessels that lead to lymph nodes (glands), where our infection-and disease-fighting white blood cells are stored. Groups of Lymph nodes are near the breast under the arm, above the collarbone, in the chest behind the breastbone, and in many other parts of the body. The lymph nodes trap bacteria, cancer cells or other harmful material.

Source National Cancer Institute

and nurses and technicians she was Adriana, the young mother who fought so hard. The woman whose arms were bruised from needles and a port and who came back week after week for experimental drugs. To them she was the woman who always had a cheerful disposition so that her little girl wouldn't be afraid.

Most Common Breast Cancers

Most breast cancers begin in the breast's milk ducts or milk-producing glands.

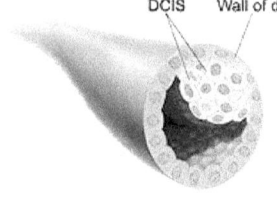

Noninvasive breast cancer (in situ) is confined to its place of origin. The most common type of noninvasive breast cancer is ductal carcinoma in situ (DCIS), located in the lining of the milk ducts.

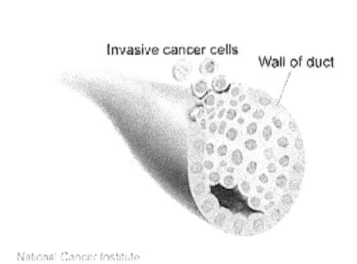

Invasive, or infiltrating breast cancer spreads from the duct or gland into surrounding tissue. Invasive ductal carcinoma (IDC), which starts in the milk duct, makes up about 70 percent of all breast cancers, and it is the type that I was diagnosed with. The second type, invasive lobular carcinoma (ILC), is less common and starts in the milk producing glands. Both types can stay near the area in the breast in which they started or spread throughout the body (metastasize) through the blood or lymph systems.

Source/Art: National Cancer Institute/Don Bliss

My parents did the best they could raising us during that difficult time. There was no Dr. Phil or Super Nanny to guide them through, and they did their best to keep the truth from hurting us. Dad initially explained Mom's illness by telling me that she got sick from the apricot danishes I used to eat with her. That only made me blame myself because I loved them and begged Mom to buy them all the time. But when she could no longer hide how deathly sick she was, Mom was candid with me. She told me she needed to see the doctor every week and that I could go with her in the ambulance. She showed me how the port in her arm worked and tried to make it fun by calling herself the Bionic Woman. She showed me her chest and said the doctors had taken the sick parts away and that it didn't hurt anymore.

My brother was younger and didn't hear most of this; they tried to protect him a little longer. There was a lot of secrecy about cancer in those days, at least in our little corner of Queens. Years later I learned that three other women in the neighborhood died from cancer when I was in grade school: the only unusual things we noticed were the funny-looking wigs they started wearing.

In spite of her nausea, fatigue and pain, Mom did everything possible to spend quality time with us during her long, drawn-out illness. She home schooled us both until we reached the first grade instead of sending us to kindergarten. She knew she was dying and she wanted us to stay home so that she could soak up every moment with us. We played games together—Candyland, jacks, Scrabble—we studied and read, and every week I wrote letters in Spanish to my grandmother in Argentina. As sick as she was, my mother made it all look effortless.

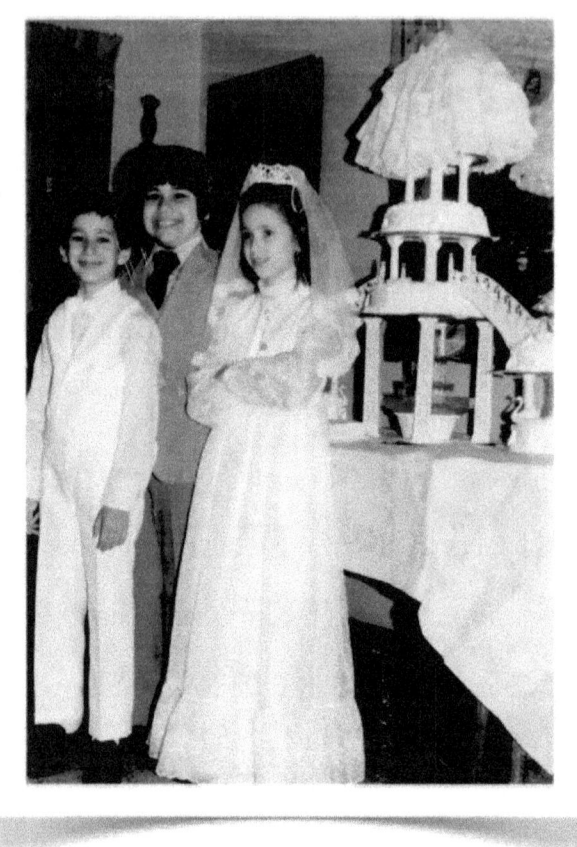

My first communion dress and cake.

One particularly bittersweet memory involves my first communion. Every girl at our church got her short white communion dress at the Queens Center Mall for $79.00, and I couldn't wait to get mine. But Mom had my dress made by a seamstress. When my big day came I was embarrassed because my dress looked like a wedding gown. I hated it. I was also mortified by the wedding cake she ordered; all the other girls celebrated with a square ice cream cake from the local shop. I had a six-tier cake with a water fountain and plastic bride on top. At only nine years old, I had never been so angry. I now appreciate that she knew it was her only chance to envision her daughter as a bride. She knew she was dying and she didn't want to miss that.

Happier memories come from the trip to Atlantic City that Mom set up for me, my brother and our Aunt Martha the summer before she died. We spent hours strolling along the boardwalk, looking out over the beach and the ocean on one side and the brightly colored shops on the other. I realized years later how difficult it must have been for her. She was green from the chemo and would throw up every ten feet or so. After the boardwalk she took us into shop after shop to buy salt-water taffy and other goodies just so she could use the "patrons only" restrooms. Mom turned a nightmarishly painful day for her into a holiday for all of us. As long as she walked the strip with us, it was a beautiful day for her. Her mind and body trumped cancer that day.

I inherited Mom's love for tradition; she never let breast cancer put a damper on birthdays, Thanksgiving or Christmas. Even when she was housebound because she was so sickly, she shopped like a madwoman from catalogs and TV shopping shows, which were just becoming popular. It's too bad that online shopping was still a few years away; she would have loved it. Now, when I binge online, I brand it as a tribute to my mother.

My friends always joked how I made cancer look glamorous. But my Mom didn't have that chance; the side effects of her chemo and the lack of drugs to help ease those side effects weren't available in her day. I, like most kids, thought my Mom walked on water. However, kids would tease me about her after she got sick. It was out of pure ignorance, but they joked about her pale green color, bad wigs or the cotton towel turban she sometimes wore on her head. The pain meds made her face look sick. Even on holidays when she put on makeup, she couldn't hide the terrible ordeal she was enduring.

On a typical day she wore a zip-up robe or other completely comfortable, wash-and-wear clothes around the house. At times I thought that it didn't seem fair that all the other Moms would pick up the kids after school, smelling and looking so nice. That used to be my Mom. After she got sick, my brother and I would walk home together from school or our Dad would pick us up. That was a small change, but to a child it's a big thing. It added to the fear about other things I didn't understand. I was

1 in 8 women in the U.S. will be diagnosed with breast cancer in their lifetime.

frightened every time they admitted her to the hospital. "What were they doing to her?" I wondered. I don't ever remember her getting her hair back after chemo. There was a little fuzz but I don't remember her hair ever coming back. She was too far gone from radiation. My Mom's hair always smelled so beautiful before she got sick. I'd hug her and her head smelled like apples or coconut. When she lost her hair we were left with the synthetic smell of her wigs.

Many of my memories of that room are not as pleasant. There were times she couldn't get up for anything, and the bedpans made me sad. She always had two or three around her room, either for vomiting or going to the toilet. There were bits of gauze and small hospital tissue boxes lying around everywhere. I was too young to know what meds she was taking, but I always counted seven bottles. Lucky seven to save my Mom. She was a guinea pig on medications, trying many kinds to combat the pain

Risk Factors That You Can CHANGE

Age and genetic characteristics are beyond your control, but other breast cancer risk factors can be lowered by your personal choices. These risks include being overweight, using hormone replacement therapy, taking birth control pills, drinking alcohol, and not having children or having your first child after age 35.

Breast Cancer Risk Factors

Certain factors have been shown to influence a woman's chance of getting breast cancer. Still, many women who develop breast cancer have no known risk factors other than growing older, and many women with known risk factors do not develop breast cancer.

A computer program called the Breast Cancer Risk Assessment Tool was developed to help doctors discuss breast cancer risk with women. For women with 0 or 1 first-degree relative (sister, mother, daughter) with breast cancer, risks increase with the age at which they deliver their first live birth, or between the ages of 25 and 29 if they do not have children. For women with 2 or more affected relatives, risks increase with age at first live birth. The tool looks at the following:

- Personal history of breast abnormalities. Two breast tissue abnormalities—ductal carcinoma in situ (DCIS) and lobular carcinoma in situ (LCIS)—are associated with increased risk for developing invasive breast cancer.
- Age. The risk of developing breast cancer increases with age. The majority of breast cancer cases occur in women older than age 50.
- Age at menarche (first menstrual period). Women who had their first menstrual period before age 12 have a slightly increased risk of breast cancer.
- Age at first live birth. Risk depends on age at first live birth and family history of breast cancer, as shown in the following table of relative risks.

Relative Risk of Developing Breast Cancer

Age at giving first live birth	# of affected relatives		
	0	1	2
20 or younger	1	2.6	6.8
20-24	1.2	2.7	5.8
25-29 or no child	1.5	2.8	4.9
30 or older	1.9	2.8	4.2

- Breast cancer among first-degree relatives (sisters, mother, daughters). Having one or more first-degree blood relatives who have been diagnosed with breast cancer increases a woman's chances of developing the disease.
- Breast biopsies. Women who have had breast biopsies have an increased risk of breast cancer, especially if the biopsy showed a change in breast tissue, known as atypical hyperplasia. These women are at increased risk because of whatever prompted the biopsies, not because of the biopsies themselves.
- Race. White women have greater risk of developing breast cancer than Black women (although Black women diagnosed with breast cancer are more likely to die of the disease).

Source: National Cancer Institute

and the side effects of chemo. Some made her feel really sick and others sedated her. It was almost like *Mommy Dearest*: because of the meds, we never knew what she was going to be like.

The nurse tried to keep a nice room, but unfortunately she covered up the smells with Lysol and rubbing alcohol. I hate the smell of cleaners to this day because it reminds me of vomit and bedpans and how sick my Mom was. It repulses me. Another smell that the nurse tried to cover over was the lingering scent of my Dad's Pall Mall reds. He never smoked in my Mom's room, but the smell followed him and permeated the place. Today we have beautiful candles that soothe the soul and perfume a room, a much nicer alternative than Lysol.

Mom's nurse, Gloria, took care of her nine to five and Mom often gave her money to buy toys for my brother and me. Mother also made sure that we had pets galore, including a dog, cats, fish and a hamster. The housekeeper couldn't keep up and my Dad was constantly cleaning up after the pets, my Mom's puke and us. He had his hands full with everything but he never complained. If he had his moments and broke down, we never saw them.

My father Joseph was completely devoted to our Mom. He pampered her, sang her songs and never stopped looking at her like she was his gorgeous bride, even after her surgeries and treatments left her frail and bald. He did everything possible to make my brother and me feel safe and loved, and he still does.

I definitely got some of my positive attitude from my Dad. For a man to stay so upbeat and patient while having so much on his plate, with no outside support or counseling like cancer family members have today, and nothing but his glass of red wine at times and his Pall Mall cigarettes to help him, he was the best husband and is still the greatest father. I also inherited his love of celebrations, and I go overboard with my birthday, just like him. Dad's birthday is in August and he starts planning it in February. Most parents don't make a fuss over their own birthdays, but not my Dad. He's 79, handsome and full of energy and life. He has worked hard to raise our family and he inspires me to be positive and thankful for everything we have. He truly loves life, travels all over the world and especially loves visiting China. He swims daily and looks about two decades younger because he finally quit smoking about 15 years ago. He lives a great, honest life, loves going to church on Sunday, loves his kids, his grandchildren; Jacqueline and James and his Labrador, Lucky.

Until his retirement, my Dad was a maitre d' at the Rainbow Room, the landmark dinner and dancing restaurant on the 65th floor of Rockefeller Center building. The owners, Patrick Daly and Tony May, were great to my Dad and very supportive of my family during my Mom's battle with cancer and beyond.

My friends kid with me today how I can be like Lucille Ball, getting myself into things. I started at an early age. My Dad wasn't very good at grounding us because we had so much heavy stuff going on with my mother, so he let us make decisions and basically do what we wanted. Super Nanny would freak at a household like ours with no set schedules, but it worked for us. Dad has had a special way of handling things. For example, one night when I was hanging out at the Rainbow Room, I went to the ladies room, where a lady hands you a towel and you can freshen up with one of several bottles of fine perfume sitting on the counter. It was the end of the night, so the room was empty, and I put all the perfume, about 10 bottles, in my book bag and took them home. When my Dad found out he said that he was disappointed in me and made me return them the next day. Most parents would put some kind of punishment like grounding on top of that, but Dad went out and bought me 10 bottles of perfume to replace the ones I had to return. One of the perfumes from that episode, Anaïs Anaïs, is still one of my favorite.

I saw my Dad work hard and love us wholeheartedly. Because of him I'm loyal, loving and a hard worker. I love traveling to beautiful places like he does. One of my most memorable trips was the one with him and my brother to Malaga, Spain, some time after my Mom died. We ate amazing foods and stayed at a wonderful hotel, and I remember ordering about 10 virgin Piña coladas or Shirley Temples a day.

My memories of visiting my Mom in the hospital are more painful than my recollections of my own stay in the hospital for cancer surgery. Everything looked so big and the atmosphere was full of uncertainty. There were fewer results and no proven track record for treating cancer back then. I remember my brother's look of horror and fright as we walked down the halls and glanced into rooms to see the old, disheveled, crabby-looking people. Everyone looked so old. "Why is our beautiful Mom in here?" we thought. The attitudes were not as personal. I don't recall any of the nurses having the compassion of those today, like the nurses who held my hand while drawing blood and used such a caring bedside manner. Instead of being afraid of things like roller coaster rides, we were fearful for our Mom in that place.

After each surgery my Mom stayed in the hospital for two weeks. She passed the time making crafts, like the small pendant she painted that I wore on a string. My Dad believed that she could hear us when she was in a coma. Years later he told me that when I spoke to her he saw tears streaming down her face, so he was sure she heard me. The day before she died I left school to visit her in the hospital. I had a feeling something was wrong. She had come out of her coma and was talking. At that moment it seemed like she was getting better. The hospital staff, however, interpreted the same thing as the clue that she was near the end. My Dad says that I asked them to leave the room because I wanted to talk to her by myself. I don't remember exactly what I said. I do remember how I felt. A wave of sadness swept over me and has blocked out the exact words we exchanged. I wanted her to know that we would be ok. My father assumed at the time that I promised her in private that I would take care of my Dad and my brother. I think that was part of it. I also wanted her to know that her love would live on in each of us.

My Mom didn't explain her mastectomy to me; every surgery was just surgery. We didn't get a real explanation of the process. My Dad was very involved—I now call him ED, effort and devotion—but I think the medical repertoire was over his head. He focused on getting her a private room and making her as comfortable as possible, but it was all new to him. He wasn't medically inclined and he was dealing with two young kids at the same time. I remember him arguing with the doctors and nurses numerous times to get her out of her discomfort; he wanted to stop the pain but he couldn't. But I don't think he even knew exactly what the surgeries entailed.

My brother, Josi (short for Joseph), who is one and a half years younger than I am, needed special attention during our Mom's illness. Boys seem to mature a little slower, so it was a lot tougher on him. My Dad was very affectionate to him, always holding him and saying, "I love you, I love you." Josi and I worried about our Mom all the time and we thought that that was the norm, that every child dealt with a sick parent. We never imagined losing her. Prior to her illness, we'd never lost anyone we loved. I'd always been very protective of my brother. We never had a "what if" conversation to talk about something happening to her and no longer having a Mom. I would let him play with his friends after school on Wednesdays, until I got home from the hospital from her chemo or radiation treatments.

Nothing can brace you for losing your Mom, but part of me seemed to know when she was near the end. One day when Mom was in the hospital I decided to skip school and take two trains by myself to visit her. Finding the route was quite a feat for a ten-year-old girl, but I got there. She woke up for awhile and talked to me. When she drifted back into her coma, I left and went home on the trains. Later that day, Dad called from the hospital to tell me that Mom had gone to sleep and would not be coming back. He told me that I should not be sad because she was at peace, and I tried to be just as comforting to Josi when I told him. But he cried and cried, and I held on to him until our Dad came home. Kids didn't have counselors at school to talk to in those days, so we kept our grief under wraps most of the time. We buried our Mom and tried to bury the pain, too.

During the funeral service at the cemetery, I became very upset when they lowered the coffin into the ground. I thought Mom was just sleeping—how could they put her into the ground? Dad made it worse by

It's Not Your Mother's Experience:
Breast Cancer Then and Now

➢ **35 Years Ago** about 75% of women diagnosed with breast cancer survived their disease at least 5 years. **TODAY** nearly 90% will survive their disease at least 5 years.

➢ **35 Years Ago** mastectomy was the only accepted surgical option for breast cancer treatment. **TODAY** breast-conserving surgery (lumpectomy) followed by local radiation therapy has replaced mastectomy as the preferred surgical approach for treating women with early stage breast cancer.

➢ **35 Years Ago** only one mammography trial for breast cancer screening had been conducted. **TODAY**, after many trials, routine mammographic screening is an accepted standard for the early detection of breast cancer.

➢ **35 Years Ago** approaches for combination chemotherapy, using multiple drugs with different mechanisms of action, for breast cancer was in its earliest stages. **TODAY** combination chemotherapy has become standard in the treatment of women with early stage breast cancer.

➢ **35 Years Ago** studies had begun on the hormonal treatment of inoperable or advanced breast cancer with tamoxifen, but had not yet been approved by the U.S. Food and Drug Administration (FDA). **TODAY** hormonal therapy is now standard for these types/stages of breast cancer. Tamoxifen and another hormone drug, raloxifene, have been shown in clinical trials to prevent the development of invasive breast cancer in women at high risk of this disease, and Tamoxifen is approved by the FDA as a breast cancer prevention drug.

➢ **35 Years Ago** scientists had not identified any genes associated with an increased risk of breast cancer. **TODAY** several breast cancer susceptibility genes have been discovered, including, BRCA1 and BRCA2, which account for about 80-90% of all hereditary breast cancers.

Source: National Cancer Institute

picking up a stick and whacking the coffin until the polished wood was covered in dents scratches. Sometime later he explained that there had been a rash of grave robberies at the time and people were digging up expensive coffins to sell them. He didn't want anyone disturbing Mom's eternal rest.

So many people loved my mother and everybody tried to be extremely nice to my brother and me at the funeral. Over and over they told us that she was going to a better place, watching over us and looking down from heaven. They wanted to comfort us, but as kids we didn't understand those phrases. The only thing I remember about those 200 people that day was that they pulled my Dad away from us and many were hugging, kissing and telling jokes. That upset me because I wanted everyone to cry and feel really terrible and maybe God would change his mind and send her back to us, and she'd wake up.

About ten of my best friends came too, and it their first time at a funeral. They were scared and felt bad. If we looked long enough at the person in the coffin we could almost see her breathing, so I swore she was going to come out of it. When I was sick and people sent so many flowers, it overwhelmed me and reminded me of her funeral. I still have the guest book, which notes that there were at least 50 big flower sprays. My Dad placed about 200 red roses over her coffin, and red roses always remind me of the day we had to say goodbye to her.

One of my friends, Eddie Laca, who would be my first boyfriend six years later, told me some funny joke at the funeral and made me laugh so hard. I thought I betrayed my mother by forgetting for a moment why I was there, and I felt terrible for a long time. Now I realize that when people get together at funerals they share their joys and their sorrows, but at the time I felt guilty for laughing. It was a confusing day in many ways, from the strange things people said to the way the 40 cars followed each other to the cemetery. I also remember when we had to go to the cemetery, I didn't understand why we had to go with 40 cars following each other, circle my house, and then go back. You didn't ask questions as a kid, you just went. I now know that the procession of cars circling our block was symbolic of my Mom coming home one last time.

After the funeral I decided I had to find a way to make us millionaires so that Dad could be on easy street and afford to hire someone to get Mom out of her grave. I still thought she was just asleep and needed some kind of expensive specialist to wake her up. I had always wanted to make my Dad proud

In 2011, there were more than 2.6 million breast cancer survivors in the US.

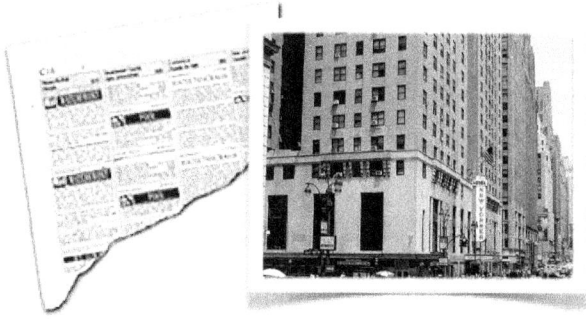

of me, and I imagined all of us together again as a rich family like the Carringtons on "Dynasty."

I was always very motivated and I came up with my first get-rich scheme one summer when we were visiting my aunt at her summer house in Spain. Her yard and garden were full of snails, and I thought that escargot cost about 100 dollars in restaurants, so I decided to collect a bunch of them to bring back to New York and sell. With the help of a neighbor girl about my age, I picked up about 200 of them, put them in a box and brought it into the kitchen. Five hours later there were snails all over the house; some of them had crawled through the dumbwaiter into other rooms. Who knew they could move so fast?

My next approach was more practical. By the time I was twelve I was growing up fast, helping my Dad with the cooking and cleaning, so I thought it was time I got a job. I looked through the classifieds in the *New York Times* and found an ad for an advertising person that paid $100,000 a year. I dressed up in my Sunday best, took the subway to 34th Street in Manhattan and walked to the Fonte & Velamonte Advertising Agency. The guy I spoke to was the sweetest person in the world; he let me sit there and pretended to give me a mini interview. He actually gave me a job in my neighborhood in Queens. At that time minimum wage was $3 an hour, but he set me to work giving out product samples at the supermarket for $10 an hour. Two products that I remember handing out were little samples of detergent and, another day, maxi pads, which were so embarrassing. My boss loves that story, showing that I was such a little go getter so young.

We didn't become millionaires with that job, but Dad eventually convinced me that Mom wasn't having the kind of sleep that she could wake from. Once I accepted that fact, I still visited her grave in the cemetery, which was nearby, but I didn't talk to Mom like she was coming back. I talked things over with her knowing that she was in a beautiful new place for good.

The cemetery didn't scare me and I never cried there. On the contrary, I was so comfortable in the setting and felt so close to her by her grave that I dreamed of getting

All women are at risk for breast cancer. Only 5-10% of those with breast cancer have inherited a mutation in the known breast cancer genes.
ACS 2010

married there. It was a serene and beautiful place. I spent many hours sitting on the grass and telling Mom stories about the people lying near her, based on the bits of information from their headstones. I told her a story about Anna, who had died at age 89 and was a nurturing and lively woman, who would watch over my Mom like a grandmother. Not far away were Albert and Lucy, who had lived a wonderful life together, raising their children, and now wanted to share all their stories with my Mom. I imagined that Mr. Mullholland, who died in 1982, was a handsome, rich actor who looked like Richard Gere and who told Mom stories with his beautiful voice. He was always by Mom's side, and I could handle that. And there was Maria, a woman who had also died young; according to her gravestone she was only 37. I told Mom she had had cancer, too, and left two little children behind. But now she danced and sang with Mom in heaven, both of them perfectly healthy and beautiful and without a care in the world. It was easy for me to handle Mom's absence imagining that all of these people were keeping her company.

I shielded Josi from the pain of being motherless as much as I could. I learned to cook and take care of him and our Dad. Most ten-year-old kids wouldn't have to go through that, but I thought it was normal.

I wanted to do it, I wanted to be like Mom's nurse, Gloria, and like a little hostess, to do things for my brother and my Dad.

* * *

What I didn't realize when I drove home from my appointment with   Dr. Kumar was how radically cancer treatment had evolved in the 25 years since Mom died. I was not in store for the kind of pain that had forced Mom to ask my brother and me to leave her room and go downstairs to watch TV with the sound turned up high. I was about to learn that chemotherapy had become much more manageable, more like coming down with the flu, and that a mastectomy no longer meant a scarred, flat chest but that plastic surgery could rebuild a woman's breasts in perfect detail, right down to the nipples. That was some of the good news to come. Fighting breast cancer wouldn't all be rosy, but it wouldn't be a death sentence either.

I spent the first two days crying at home. My closest friends sat with me, consoling me with their presence. There were no appropriate words to say. Each of them had a busy life. We usually had to schedule our socializing weeks in advance and never saw each other as much as we wanted to, but they didn't hesitate to make time for me when a crisis hit. I looked around the living room and wondered if the next time they would all be together would be at my funeral. I loved my life so much. I wanted more life and happiness. I knew I needed to get all the tears out so that I could start fighting and make sure my friends wouldn't go to my funeral until they were old and gray.

It would take a few days to release my fears and shake off my self-pity. What if it was actually my time? In 2001 I had survived a terrible car accident that had put me in bed for three months, followed by a full year of painful physical therapy. The doctors said my foot bones were so crushed that I would walk with a limp for the rest of my life. Michael had to carry me to the bathroom and feed me. It was awful, but I put every ounce of strength into my physical therapy and I won. I don't have a limp. I learned that life is worth fighting for, and I had to get ready to put that belief to the test again.

What made me finally get ready for the biggest battle yet? The same thing that had filled me with the most fear when I got my diagnosis, the memory of my Mom. She endured brutal surgeries and treatments, but she never gave up. My recovery from the car accident proved to me that I had inherited her courage, and I began to feel a warm glow of hope where the darkness had been.

80 % of all lumps found in the breast turn out to be benign.

My Dad and brother needed more time to process my diagnosis. They were beside themselves. The thought of losing me was too much and they wanted to take all the pain and decision making away. When I was growing up, Dad could make everything alright with his songs, with our trips to the Plaza Hotel for clams and Shirley Temples, with elevator rides up to the Rainbow Room for bowls of tartufo. He knew he had always been my hero, but that he couldn't slay my dragons now.

There were so many things I still wanted to do, so many people I loved and so much I wanted to live for. I didn't have a choice. Fighting was the only option, so I dusted myself off and got ready.

Looking back on my journey with breast cancer, from my diagnosis to my last chemotherapy treatment, I know that the experience made me stronger physically, mentally and spiritually. I understand the power of all the love in my life and have a new set of priorities. I have been given a second chance, and I am grateful for everything in my life, just as it is. As a breast cancer survivor, I can truly say that the grass is always greener on my side.

❖ Tell every woman you know that early detection can save her life! Women in the United States get breast cancer more than any other type of cancer except skin cancer, and it is the second cause of cancer death in American women next to lung cancer. Make it a habit to do a breast self-exam every month—the best time is right after your period, when your breasts are the least swollen or tender. A detailed, step-by-step guide to the self exam can be found on the Mayo Clinic website at www.mayoclinic.com/health/ breast-self-exam/WO00026.

❖ Become familiar with your breasts every month so that you can easily detect any changes that should immediately be checked out by your doctor, such as:

–lumps or lumpiness

–changes in size

–puckering or dimpling

–areas of thickened tissue

–pulling in of the nipple or a discharge from the nipple

–unusual or unexplained pain.

Lumps or thickening could be caused by hormonal changes during your period, a fibrous lump called a fibroadenoma, fluid-filled cysts, small calcium spots or star-shaped abnormalities called radial scars.

❖ A list of conventional mammography facilities is available by calling the Cancer Information Service at 1–800–4–CANCER (1–800–422–6237), or by visiting the FDA Web site at http://www.accessdata.fda.gov/scripts/cdrh/cfdocs/cfMQSA/ mqsa.cfm.

❖ Reach out for support from your friends and family.

I found comfort and encouragement from my personal support system as well as music, movies, books and poetry, including this poem by Brian Gil:

Hang in There, Hold On, and
Keep Your Spirits Up!

If you ever need some extra encouragement ➔If you would like to be reminded once in a while that you're so special ➔I want you to remember this . . . and I hope it brings you a smile ➔Never forget what a treasure you are ➔Try to realize how important you are in the eyes of my world ➔No matter where you go, my hopes and my heart travel beside you every step of the way ➔And I know, even though difficulties come to everyone, it isn't fair when they hang around longer than they should ➔If I could wish the clouds away, the welcoming breeze of a brand- new day would warm your life right this very minute ➔But until a new days comes along, I know that you'll always be strong enough to see things through . . .

I have so much faith in you ➔I know how much strength and courage you have inside ➔ I know you can find all the patience it takes ➔You can turn to the times in the past when challenges were met, when you survived, when you were rewarded with success, and when you learned to believe in so much within

you ➜ *You have so much going for you, and I know*
that you're going to see your way through anything
that comes along ➜ *I know that brighter days are*
going to find a way to shine in your windows and
chase away any blues ➜ *And of all the things I am*
most certain of . . . I know that no one deserves more
smiles, success, friendship, or love

. . . than the special person I see

every time I look at you ➜

(Brian Gil, *Hang in There—Life Can be Hard*
Sometimes, But It's Going to be Okay, Blue Mountain
Arts, 2004)

Chapter 2

Searching for Dr. Right

"Ultimately we know deeply that the other side of
every fear is a freedom."

—Marilyn Ferguson

The fear that set in after I heard my diagnosis was based on the memory of what breast cancer did to my mother. The core of this fear was the most basic one of all: death. For me, death had come too soon for my Mom. But my knowledge of her experience had a positive effect as well. She had shown me her mastectomy scars not to try to gain pity, but to teach me that some battles leave scars, and every battle that keeps us alive and with our loved ones is a battle worth fighting. I knew that the first step in my fight to stay alive was to teach myself about every detail of current breast cancer treatment.

Doctors, nurses, friends and colleagues had the best intentions in mind when they offered advice, but I needed a thorough crash course that covered each issue, from surgical options to alternative treatments. What were the criteria for choosing between partial and complete breast removal? How natural looking was breast reconstruction? What were the best medications to take to make chemotherapy as painless as possible? What alternative therapies worked best to enhance recovery from surgery and to help build up my strength during chemotherapy?

Knowledge is definitely power, and understanding all the options *I used knowledge as a tool to break away from fear and panic . . .* would not only lessen my fear but also empower me to get through every phase of my treatment with the positive outlook that is so critical for healing.

The first issue I set out to research was breast surgery and I took a very pro-active approach. The decision to remove only part of the breast, one breast or both is a very personal choice for every woman facing breast cancer. Some women prefer a lumpectomy because they will preserve one breast, undergo less surgery and have a shorter recovery time. But there is also a significant chance for reoccurrence, which would mean going through the entire process again. The decision is also complicated by our emotional reaction to losing this part of our body.

. . . so I urge you to be proactive and stick to the facts!

I was blessed with nice-sized, perky breasts. I remember like yesterday my first Victoria's Secret black-and-gold bikini. I always loved being a woman, wearing beautiful clothes and swimsuits and pampering myself. It's a mystery how I became such a girlie girl growing up without a mother; I didn't have sisters to play dress-up with and my Dad had to buy me my first bra. Like most young women, my love of pretty clothes and fascination with my growing-up body also had a shadow side. As beautiful as I felt most times, there was also a feeling of inadequacy about my body image. Should I be thinner, taller, have bigger breasts? I guess we are never satisfied with what we have until we are faced with losing it entirely. When I started researching breast surgery options, I had to overcome my resistance to making this decision in the first place. I didn't want to change a thing on me. I sure didn't want to lose my breasts!

That was the time to get tough. I needed to start acting more like my gynecologist, Lisa Eng, whom I selected when I signed on for health benefits at work. She had been recommended by a friend at work who knew that we had both gone to Queens College. Meeting Dr. Eng for the first

I dove into the process by talking to breast cancer survivors, medical professionals, people at work and also doing my homework on the web.

21 Questions to Ask Your Breast Surgeon and Oncologist

1. What is the prognosis? Cure rate?

2. Am I at high risk for the cancer to come back?

3. What stage of breast cancer do I have?

4. How many breast cancer surgeries have you done?

5. How large will my scar be? Where will it be?

6. How much breast tissue will be removed?

7. What are my chances of lymphedema [swelling of the lymph vessels or nodes]?

8. How many surgeries will I need?

9. Do I need chemotherapy?

10. Will I need radiation and how do you determine this?

11. How will chemotherapy affect my heart?

12. What are the risks and benefits of chemotherapy?

13. How long will I need chemotherapy?

14. Can I work during chemotherapy?

15. What drugs do you recommend?

16. Lymph node involvement: Can it spread to other parts of my body?

17. What is the size of the tumor?

18. What is the grade of my cancer?

19. Should I have additional imaging, such as an MRI?

20. How long will my recovery take?

21. Insurance: How much is covered?

time was an experience. She is a major figure in the New York Asian community, a primary physician as well as gynecologist with a busy practice. She is one of the strongest and brightest people I know, but at our first appointment she struck me as way off the mark. I said that I wanted children, and she told me straight out to get pregnant as soon as I could, then get rid of my breasts and ovaries. I thought she was nuts; I was 25 and in fantastic shape. My grandmother was in her late sixties, cancer-free and fabulous. Doctor Eng came across as aggressive, insensitive and radical, and I left her office without taking her seriously.

But facing breast cancer turned me around, quick. I had to get radical like Dr. Eng, so I started out by working up a strategy for choosing a breast surgeon. I dove into the process by talking to breast cancer survivors, medical professionals, people at work and also doing my homework on the web. Based on all of this research, I made up a short list of the top breast surgeons in the New York area. I knew their backgrounds and experience, but that wasn't enough. I made appointments to see each of them personally so that I could evaluate them face to face. In a decision this important, I wasn't going to leave my instincts out of it. I needed to be comfortable with the person who was going to carve out my cancer.

After meeting with everyone on my list, I factored in all the information— including my gut feelings—and chose Michael Osborne at Cornell. Each doctor I met had impressive credentials, track records and expertise, but Dr. Osborne was the most comforting. He talked to me with the care and genuine concern of a father giving life-or-death advice to his daughter. From the outset, he was compassionate yet very straightforward.

Doctor Osborne believed strongly in breast preservation. He firmly recommended that I have a lumpectomy because, as I was only 34, he thought that time was on my side. By this time, however, I had been leaning heavily toward having a double mastectomy instead of some type of breast-sparing surgery. I didn't want to revisit this dark place, and I was starting to believe there was no other option for me.

After sharing these thoughts with Dr. Osborne, he insisted I meet with a psychiatrist three times over the course of the next week. The psychiatrist he sent me to specializes in oncology, and she worked hard to persuade me to have a lumpectomy. She focused on the fact that I could regret losing both breasts and that this could lead to other issues. I appreciated her efforts, but

Make informed decisions by finding a BALANCE between official medical information and the experiences of individual cancer survivors.

throughout each session I thought, "lady, one breast is not better than two. You don't know how traumatizing it is to live with the memory of your mother's losing battle with this terrible disease." The prospect of feeling regret down the line didn't measure up to the prospect of losing my life to another incidence of cancer. After three visits, I had another appointment with Dr. Osborne to tell him I still wasn't convinced about the lumpectomy. He understood, but he also went back over the benefits of taking the easiest possible course. It was clear that he didn't want me to endure unnecessary emotional and psychological baggage in the future. I was comforted by that, but I still wasn't sold on the idea.

I decided that I needed to hear about some real-life outcomes in order to make my decision, and I set out to talk to as many breast cancer survivors I could find. Fortunately, my work made me familiar with a lot of doctors, and many of them asked their patients if they'd be willing to talk to me. As a result, I spoke to 75 women. My homegrown research study had a big impact on my decision. Some of the women I talked to had chosen to have lumpectomies and others had undergone bilateral mastectomies. One woman had a lumpectomy the first time and, when the cancer returned, opted for a mastectomy. The major difference was the peace of mind of those who had taken the more drastic route. Each of

Genetic Testing for Breast Cancer

About 5 to 10 percent of women diagnosed with breast cancer have a hereditary form of the disease. Changes, called alterations or mutations, in certain genes make some women more susceptible to developing breast and other types of cancer. Inherited alterations in the genes called BRCA1 and BRCA2 (short for breast cancer 1 and breast cancer 2) are involved in many cases of hereditary breast and ovarian cancer. Researchers are searching for other genes that may also increase a woman's cancer risk.

BRCA1 is a gene that normally helps to suppress cell growth. A person who inherits a mutated (changed) BRCA1 gene has a higher risk of getting breast, ovarian, or prostate cancer.

BRCA2 is a another gene that normally helps to suppress cell growth. A person who inherits a mutated (changed) BRCA2 gene has a higher risk of getting breast, ovarian, or prostate cancer.

Type of Cancer	Percent of General Population That Will Develop Disease	Percent of Those With BRCA1 Mutation Who Will Develop Disease	Percent of Those With BRCA2 Mutation Who Will Develop Disease
Breast	12.5%	55% to 85%	33% to 86%
Ovarian	1.43%	28% to 44%	10% to 30%
Prostate	4.5 to 6.0%	12% to 18%	12% to 18%
Male Breast Cancer	Less than 1%	6%	4% to 14%
Pancreatic	0.6%	n.a.	6% to 7%

Source for Table: Genetic Health, www.genetichealth.com/
brovgen_of_brov_cancer.shtml

them stressed the fact that after being diagnosed with breast cancer you are extensively monitored the first five years for recurrence. The chance of cancer showing up again is high enough that many women opt for a double mastectomy, which eliminates all the fear and increases the chances for a long, happy life. The chief complaint I heard from the women who chose to have a lumpectomy was that their breasts weren't symmetrical. One was perfect—the saline or silicone implant—and the other hung lower. This deeply affected some of them. When you jump out of the shower every day and see this dramatic imbalance it takes a toll on your self-esteem. These women helped me realize that cancer already takes a part of your body and soul—why let it steal more? That made sense, but there would be more factors to weigh before making my decision.

Talking to breast cancer survivors did more than give me a close look at surgical options for breast surgery. Meeting them and witnessing their healthy lives gave me hope and helped me

You Cannot Be Denied Insurance or Employment Over Your BRAC Gene Testing Results

A new law, the Genetic Information Nondiscrimination Act (GINA) of 2008, protects people from genetic discrimination by health insurers or employers.

look beyond the treatments I was about to undergo and imagine a bright future. One of them, Elaine, the wife of one of my long-time clients, became a mother figure for me by explaining the mastectomy process, giving advice about what to look for in doctors and hospitals. She went to some of my appointments with me. On her own she was very comforting and reassuring, and seeing her with her husband was even more encouraging. Both in their 60s, they acted like teenagers in love. Her doctor husband melted when he looked at her and told me that he was going to take her shoe shopping. Elaine and her husband gave me hope that relationships can survive breast cancer and that there are good men out there. Breast cancer is not the end.

Doctor Osborne wanted me to have as much information as possible to help in my decision, so he scheduled genetic testing to find out if I had inherited an altered breast cancer gene. The chances of having the abnormal gene are high if a woman has two or more close family members who have had breast or ovarian cancer, and I fit that category. Relatives considered close family members include one's mother, father, sister, brother, grandparent on either side, as well as mother and father's siblings. My mother's sister, Martha, got breast cancer at roughly the same time my mother did. She completely changed her life when she got her diagnosis because she didn't want her family to know, especially her mother, who was already losing one daughter to the disease. Aunt Martha had always been a free spirit and a rebel, so it wasn't hard for her to pick up and move to another country and start a new life.

For years the family thought she had moved to Israel just for a change, so when my mother died Dad mailed Martha photos from the funeral, thinking she would be glad to be included. Eventually we learned that Martha had had a lumpectomy and recovered physically and emotionally without any family or friends around her. Today, she's very healthy and also fanatic about her daughter having regular mammograms and taking every precaution. Samantha, my first cousin, got tested for alterations in her Breast Cancer Gene 1 (BRCA1) and Gene 2 (BRCA2), and came up negative.

My results weren't as good; my BRCA1 test was positive and I was a high risk for both breast and ovarian cancer. This clinched my decision about having a double mastectomy, and Dr. Osborne changed his mind, too. Unfortunately, genetic testing isn't the last word in diagnosis. I was shocked to learn that the majority of women who get breast cancer don't have a family history and don't have the altered genes. That's why

Three Types of Breast Surgery

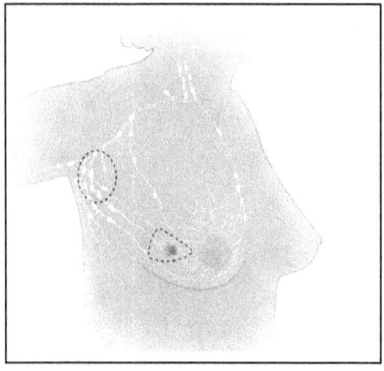

In BREAST-SPARING SURGERY, the surgeon removes the tumor in the breast and some tissue around it. Lymph nodes under the arm may also be removed, as well as some of the lining over the chest muscles below the tumor.

In TOTAL (SIMPLE) MASTECTOMY, the surgeon removes the whole breast. Some lymph nodes under the arm may also be removed.

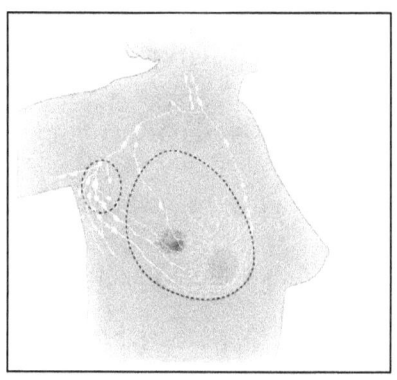

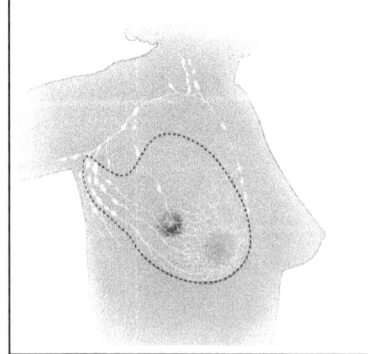

In MODIFIED RADICAL MASTECTOMY, the surgeon removes the whole breast and most or all of the lymph nodes under the arm. Often, the lining over the chest muscles is removed. A small chest muscle also may be taken out to make it easier to remove the lymph nodes.

Source/Art: National Cancer Institute/

Don Bliss

women like my aunt Martha are adamant about telling all the women they know about the importance of getting yearly mammograms.

By choosing to lose both of my breasts I gave myself the best chance of enjoying a long, healthy life. I wasn't thinking cosmetically. Truly, at that point I didn't care what my body would look like. The end result was a clean bill of health, and that's all that mattered. I wasn't resentful that I had cancer. I wanted to do everything possible to ensure my survival and have years of memories. Small everyday problems were no longer relevant, and I even stopped worrying about carrying a big Zorro scar on my chest. My boyfriend, Michael, shared my view that being alive would be more than enough. We were grateful that I was going to be ok. The choice seemed clear: my breasts or my life. I chose life. Little did I know at the beginning of this decision process that breast surgery had made big advances since my mother's day and that reconstructive surgery could give me a new pair of beautiful and natural-looking breasts.

I soon learned that today's medical advances allow women facing a double mastectomy to look forward to a body just as attractive — maybe even more so — at the end of their ordeal. I didn't have to sacrifice my breasts permanently. State-of-the-art post-cancer reconstruction methods promised me the best of both worlds — low odds for cancer recurrence and a whole, healthy body.

Doctor Osborne explained that during the mastectomy he would remove the cancer, and then my plastic surgeon would remove the breast tissue and save as much skin as possible for the breast reconstruction. So the reconstruction process would begin immediately, and I needed to find a plastic surgeon before I could schedule the mastectomy. Using the same approach I had designed to find Dr. Osborne, I began a new round of research to find a plastic surgeon with the combination of skill and nurturing that had made Dr. Osborne such an excellent choice.

It was tough to face the idea of spending so much time and energy researching plastic surgeons at that point. Part of me was still in shock over what was happening. Another part was preoccupied with rearranging my life to make time for recovering from surgery and going through chemotherapy. I could have taken the easy route and signed on with the plastic surgeon Dr. Kumar recommended the same day he gave me my diagnosis. But this was a decision about my body, my feminine identity, my life, and I wasn't about to start taking shortcuts. Besides, I had already met with that plastic surgeon and from the first moment I sat in his office I knew he wasn't the one. As a matter of fact, I couldn't stand him. So I had my work cut out for me.

Going back to my friends, relatives and business associates to ask for their opinions about plastic surgeons didn't seem out of line. They had been so helpful in my search for a breast surgeon that I figured they would have some good leads this time, too, and I didn't think they would mind. After all, we ask each other for recommendations of restaurants, shopping, hair stylists, a contractors and dentist, right? What is more important than asking for help to get the best results for a life-changing medical procedure? There's no time to be shy when it comes to getting the medical specialists who are a perfect fit for you and your situation.

Plastic surgery is a glamorous profession. Some physicians in the field let their celebrity go to their heads and become arrogant and very insensitive. I should have known that I would come across a few like that. It was a shocking experience at times. The first doctor walked into the exam room, talked to me about generalities for about three minutes, then grabbed a marker and started writing on my

Ask your current doctor, friends and breast cancer survivors to recommend a breast surgeon. Once you have chosen this specialist, ask whom he/she recommends for a plastic surgeon.

chest. He said that he would cut here, remove there, et cetera, as if I were a blackboard. I felt terrible about myself and left his office feeling scared stiff. By the time I got home I was more angry than afraid. I was facing the removal of both of my breasts, and a little empathy, a little compassion wasn't asking too much.

But compassion doesn't equate with being a great surgeon. He or she can be highly successful by racking up a lot of great outcomes and leaving the good bedside manner out of it. Some surgeons I met treated everyone badly. While sitting in the waiting room to meet another doctor on my list, I heard him yell at a nurse and another woman on his staff. I was already nervous, and his unprofessional outburst made me feel horrible. The last thing I needed was to feel sorry for his staff and angry at him. Keeping up with my search took a lot of energy, but I insisted on finding a surgeon with a mix of compassion and skill. Don't get me wrong, credentials are important. I am sure the doctors I didn't choose probably blessed and saved a lot of people. But I promised myself that I would only work with someone whose heart was really in the work.

After a few more unsatisfying visits to offices across Brooklyn and Queens, I found myself running out of time and asked Dr. Osborne for an opinion. He recommended one of his colleagues at Cornell, Gregory

LaTrenta. I took my friend Daisy to my first meeting with Dr. LaTrenta, and we were both extremely nervous as we waited for him to come into his office. What if he turned out to be a schmuck like so many of the other plastic surgeons I'd met? He walked in, introduced himself, sat down and looked at my file. As he read, a very sad look fell across his face. After a few minutes he looked up and said he couldn't believe that one of the young women sitting in front of him was so ill and was going to be his patient. I broke down in tears and told him I was the one.

In the exam room, Dr. LaTrenta did an initial examination and told me that I had nice breasts but that they were not healthy. "I am going to give you beautiful and healthy breasts," he said. After talking to me for nearly an hour, answering all my questions and explaining the procedures in detail, he completely erased all my fears about the surgery.

Before and after my reconstructive surgery, Dr. LaTrenta's staff was very compassionate and informative as well. Olivia, his front-office receptionist, always had a smile when I walked in and she ran around the counter to hug me. Nicole, the nurse, always had practical and up-to-date recommendations about creams for scar removal, what to wear to stay comfortable

Be strong, positive and pick a great doctor and you'll have beautiful, healthy breasts

How to Choose Your Breast Reconstruction Surgeon

by Gregory LaTrenta, M.D. P.C, F.A.C.S

There are several very important criteria that must be satisfied when choosing a plastic and reconstructive surgeon.

First and foremost is making certain the surgeon is board certified in plastic surgery. The American Board of Medical Specialists has recently redesignated "plastic and reconstructive surgery" to "plastic surgery." This is not be confused with facial plastic surgery, opthalmoplastic surgery, or cosmetic surgery, designations that apply to ENT, ophthalmology and dermatology sub-specialties, respectively.

Second, the plastic surgeon you choose should devote a substantial portion of his or her practice to breast reconstruction and not be what is colloquially called a "dabbler."

Thirdly, this breast surgeon and the plastic surgeon should have an excellent working relationship in order to optimize your care. By definition, an excellent working relationship means that they work frequently with one another, publish peer-reviewed articles together and have a deep abiding respect for one another. Other important factors include interviewing previous patients, reviewing the doctor's photos of patients who have undergone breast reconstruction and, most important, having a sense of trust in the doctor you've chosen.

during recovery and where to find pretty and flattering mastectomy bras (to replace the ugly ones that the hospital gives you.) Another person in the office, Johnette, was a beautiful person inside and out. She helped me with billing and insurance questions and worked out a payment plan for my out-of-pocket costs. She treated me like a family member, not a business transaction. If the doctor was running late they called me so that I wouldn't waste my time in the waiting room, which made me feel like my time really mattered to them. Each staff person became part of my support system and acted like a therapist, cheering me on and giving me compliments. That kind of attention really blew me away. I'm a drug rep, so I'm in doctors' offices almost every day, and I rarely see that kind of nurturing. If you take the time to look, you can find a surgeon and office staff that put you first, too.

Daisy was so taken with everything and felt so positive about Dr. LaTrenta that before he left the exam room she asked him about getting a breast lift. We laughed about that, but when he left the room Daisy and I hugged each other and I started crying again. After all the gray exam rooms, cold hands and hard egos I'd gone through in my search for a plastic surgeon, my path led me to one of the most warm, encouraging and all-around great people I'd ever met. It was all worth the effort. I wasn't even scheduled for surgery yet, but I knew that Dr. LaTrenta was a godsend who would make all the difference.

Sometimes, we rush into things because we feel we have no other choice, we lack time or we do not know any better. In any serious matter, be sure about who or what you choose. I have no regrets with any of my physicians or treatment options. And if you are unsure about something important, even after you have done your homework. Surround yourself with people who are knowledgeable and can help.

Tips

To find the breast surgeon, plastic surgeon and oncologist who is perfect for you, educate yourself:

- ❖ Participate in online breast cancer chats and discussion groups.

- ❖ Follow through by obtaining suggested articles, books, support groups and organizations.

- ❖ Listen to, read or download prerecorded personal stories and discussions among breast cancer survivors and caregivers.

- ❖ Find and communicate with other survivors and caregivers. Your primary care physician may be a good place to get your first referrals. Invite survivors to communicate with you in the way that is most comfortable for them: phone, email or in person.

Chapter 3

On the Table

"You gain strength, courage, and confidence by
every experience in which you really stop to look
fear in the face. You must do the thing which you
think you cannot do."

—Eleanor Roosevelt

On April 5, 2005, the night before my surgery, Daisy came over and took

pictures of my breasts. She meant well by offering me something to

remember them by, but it didn't make me any less horrified of what was to

come. I was not proud of how frightened I was. Doctor LaTrenta had put

me completely at ease about how beautiful, natural looking and healthy

the final outcome was going to be. When it came right down to it however

I was still facing major surgery in a few hours and when I woke afterward

my breasts would be gone.

I kept thinking about how many times I'd been critical of my body and how I'd give anything to take it all back to stay exactly the same. I was me and I was perfect. I was scared to death to lose what made me feminine.

Later that evening Anne and I met up with a bunch of my friends for dinner at Abbracamiento's in Middle Village, Queens, one of my favorite neighborhood restaurants. The family that owns the place, John, Joseph, and Marie, always make their customers feel special and it was exactly the kind of attention I needed that night. I finished off a porterhouse steak, baked clams, sausage and cannolis for dessert, all before midnight, to keep within the rules for surgery the next morning. A few times I stopped to think how surreal it was this was the last time we'd be all be out eating together with things as they were. The next time everything would be different. I would be different, forever. But for the moment I felt great, looked great, didn't want pity and just reveled in the love and attention. My friends supported me, toasted me and we shared a lot laughs.

Back at home, my boyfriend Michael held me all night. I knew that he was very scared as well. He tried to be as

"We cannot discover new oceans unless we have the courage to lose sight of the shore."
—André Gide

brave as he possibly could, but he had never lost anyone close to him and I knew he was frightened. It didn't help that I kept asking questions What if I have a bad reaction to the anesthesia? Could I have a heart attack during my surgery? Will you help give away my things if I don't make it? Earlier that afternoon I had visited my best friend, Claudia, and her husband, Sal, who is a lawyer, so that I could draw up my will. Ever since the attacks of 9/11 I had thought about the importance of having a will, so I asked Sal to do that for me before I had my surgery. It was very disturbing for them to have to deal with this and act as witnesses to the document. I was only 33 years old and they had known me as such a positive person with so much joy for life that it was a tough thing for them to digest. It was a morbid moment. That night I cried myself to sleep, and four hours later the alarm went off.

The morning started out with more questions. Why was I going to the hospital? I felt healthy, could this be happening to me. I had four opinions from four different doctors, but could there still be a chance for error? Only time would tell how the rest of my life would go. Doctor Osborne would either isolate the tumor and I would be okay, or it could be the beginning of the end.

At the hospital, standing barefoot in the freezing changing room, I knew there was no turning back. I slipped on a surgical gown and tucked my long hair into a hairnet. The clonopine I took an hour earlier was helping me relax. I was the first surgery on the schedule, and my stomach was growling. At least on death row they feed you good before the inevitable, I thought.

I prayed to God to give me a sign that it was going to be okay. I received it a minute later when I saw Dr. Alviva Preminger in the operating room. She is the daughter of one of my physician customers and her name means "life." That was my sign that I was going to get through this just fine. Dr. Preminger is a lovely woman, inside and out, and she was doing her breast surgery rotation with Dr. Osborne. As a urology drug representative at a pharmaceutical company, I knew a lot of urologists but rarely met doctors in other disciplines. What were the chances I would know the resident rotating in breast surgery at this hospital? The anesthesiologist put an IV line in my arm and Alviva held my hand until I fell asleep.

After seven hours of surgery the nurses rolled me into the recovery room. Doctor LaTrenta had placed two tissue expanders beneath the skin where my breasts had been. Over the next three months he would gradually fill them with saline so that the breast skin would expand and eventually become large enough to hold two permanent breast implants.

I woke up to see my best friend Ivette at my side, holding my hand and lightly touching my face. My first sensation was joy—I was exhausted but ecstatic to be breathing and alive. There was no pain because I was on a morphine drip. I didn't care that the surgeons had removed both of my breasts. I was alive! I immersed myself in the wonderful spirit of oxygen and life.

The morphine and exhaustion left me so dizzy that I was grateful for the catheter that allowed me to stay in bed. It was supposed to be removed shortly after surgery, but I pleaded with the nurse to leave it in an extra day. Soon after I was moved to my room Dr. Osborne came in and was pleased to report no lymph nodes were involved. They were clean. This meant that the recovery process would be much easier and less complicated. Dad and my friend Denise were in the room, and they cried for joy. I looked at them, felt their love for me, and realized how ironic it is that life deals you a deck of cards like this and then turns it into good fortune, the good fortune of appreciating every piece of good news, every precious moment of life.

That first night after surgery Michael crawled into my hospital bed and slept with me through the night. I felt so secure to have him there with me. I was uncomfortable and extremely fatigued, but I wasn't in any pain. I squeezed the morphine drip button every ten minutes.

The next day the nurses removed my catheter and wouldn't let me rest until I had gotten out of bed and walked around. Then my friend Claudia stopped by and did my makeup. I knew I'd feel better when my family and friends came to visit if I looked more like my old self instead of pale and washed out. It sounds like a little thing, but it helped me feel more in control. When I looked in the mirror, I thought I looked great. My hair was messy in a sexy way. I really didn't feel different. I felt like the tumor that could kill me was out and I would put Humpty Dumpty back together again.

I couldn't look at my chest yet, though. Michael and some of my girlfriends did, and no one looked horrified. They were all able to look me straight in the eye and swear it wasn't too bad considering all my breast tissue was gone. Michael is extremely squeamish and even he was okay. I would have drains in for three weeks before starting the tissue expansion.

Ivette spoiled me because she was a physical therapist at Cornell, which was a happy coincidence, and was able to stop in my room several

71

times a day. We've been best friends since childhood, so having her close right after surgery made me feel right at home. She stocked the refrigerator in my room with my favorite beverages, Orangina and Perrier, and brought in my favorite blanket, pillow, socks and pictures from home.

Another friend, Anne, brought me one of my favorite desserts, a cake made up of about twenty thin crepe layers and a creamy filling, from a cake boutique in Manhattan. I ate three slices but regretted it an hour later when the nausea kicked in. Solid foods, especially sweets, are not the best thing to indulge in after surgery and anesthesia. Thankfully, a nurse came to the rescue with a neat trick to combat the nausea—salty potato chips! A healer after my own heart. I knew there were more surgeries to follow, as well as chemotherapy, but moments like those kept me living in the moment and feeling grateful for every kind act.

During my three-day recovery in the hospital, I felt very carefree and at peace with no worries or concerns. I felt really great. Sitting on my hospital bed, I looked across the room into the mirror and still felt like the old me. All bandaged up, I didn't sense that my breasts were missing and there was no pain. By the third day I was ready to leave. Insurance would probably have paid for another two days, but I had the doctors' permission to be discharged and I wanted out. Michael packed me up and got me home that Friday afternoon. Most breast cancer survivors I talk to say that they stayed longer than three days, but I was so happy to be alive and feeling good that I couldn't wait to get home. I had thought I was going to die and then I woke up surrounded by all of my loved ones—I was ecstatic.

When I was released from the hospital, my family and friends continued to give me the love and support that had made such a big difference every day of my recovery. One job was to care for the Jackson-Pratt, or JP drains at home. Even though Michael and I are both squeamish, we didn't have any problem with the drains. I probably could have managed very well on my own, but Michael, Ivette and my brother made up a schedule to come over and help change them. The suction-bulb drains continuously pulled fluid from my chest area as the surgical wounds healed, and they needed to be emptied two to three times a day. I attached the plastic bulbs to my clothing with a safety pin to make sure it would not pull on the tubing, and it was a lot simpler than I thought it would be. We measured the drainage each time we emptied the bulbs, and when there was less than 30cc's in a 24-hour period the JP's were ready to come out. So far, so good.

Bilateral Mastectomy
Surgical Removal of Both Breasts:
A Matter of Choice

by Gregory LaTrenta, M.D. P.C, F.A.C.S.

For a large variety of reasons, more patients, and especially younger patients, are requesting bilateral mastectomy and bilateral breast reconstruction using gel silicone implants. The reasons for this are numerous. Reconstructive surgeons have raised the bar so to speak on breast reconstructive results, making bilateral breast reconstruction a much more attractive option for patients facing the shadow of breast cancer. Scars are smaller, recovery is more rapid, and reconstructive surgery is immediate after the mastectomy. Genetic testing has also become an integral predicative tool for patients with a family history of breast cancer and for those patients of Ashkenazi heritage. Genetic testing studies have been shown that the genes have overwhelming penetrance [the frequency with which a gene produces its effect] for the disease.

Gel silicone breast prostheses are now FDA-approved medical devices, lifting the fear many patients have had of these devices in the past. Gel silicone manufacturers have also offered implants in more varied shapes and sizes than ever before as breast implant surgery has skyrocketed to the number-one plastic surgical procedure performed since the FDA approved the devices. And although mastectomy patients have similar survival rates compared to women who have had lumpectomy performed, many mastectomy patients feel that their survival is of far greater quality. Mastectomy patients no longer need mammograms of the affected breast, so they are no longer plagued with the dreaded anxiety of a possible cancer recurrence every time they have mammography performed. And unlike lumpectomy and radiation patients, immediate breast reconstruction patients do not require long and involved flap procedures, many of which have inherent risks and prolonged recovery times. All of these factors have greatly reduced the number of mastectomy patients who opt for flap reconstruction, and have greatly increased the number of patients opting for bilateral implant reconstruction.

In four sessions over the next several weeks, Dr. LaTrenta inflated my tissue expanders with saline solution. These procedures were scheduled between chemotherapy treatments, and I'll never forget the state I was in when I showed up at my first expander appointment. I had taken too many painkillers after reading <u>I Wore Lipstick to My Mastectomy</u> by Geralyn Lucas. She sensationalized it to sell books and it put the fear of God in me. She described her tissue expander appointments as real nightmares: "I should have worn a hard hat. Expanding is a polite way of saying that your plastic is going to pull your skin so hard that you'll want to scream 'motherfucker!' as loud as you can." Passages like that unraveled my common sense and took me back a few steps, so I overmedicated to prepare myself. My girlfriend Dawn drove me to the appointment because I was, let's just say, too *comfortable* to get there on my own.

I didn't feel a thing as Dr. LaTrenta and his nurse Jennifer worked on me. It took about ten minutes. I looked and touched and I was still flat as a wall. I said, "more, please." They laughed, but didn't give me any more. The skin must be stretched very gradually in order to stay healthy. It felt awkward to be so flat,

> *A tissue expander is like an inflatable breast implant and the process of expansion can take several weeks.*

but tissue expansion is worth the wait because the skin is a perfect match and there is little scarring. Because the skin is intact, instead of harvested from another part of the body, there's very little risk that it will die because it is attached to its normal blood and nerve supply. Tissue expansion could be called "growing your breasts back..." at least part of them.

On August 30th, nearly five months after my mastectomy, I went in for my second reconstructive surgery, mammoplasty replacement. The tissue expanders had worked perfectly and my breast skin was ready to take cohesive silicone implants.

After Breast Surgery:
- *Stay optimistic and mentally strong*
- *Avoid heavy lifting*
- *Stretch and exercise to help regain your range of motion.*
- *See a physical therapist to help you with mobility*

Again, I didn't jump into the decision to choose silicone over saline. I polled several women and found that the women who chose saline switched to silicone implants about six months to a year later because of the disturbing swishing sounds. Each felt like she had a waterbed strapped to her chest. This was due to their lack of breast tissue—women who have silicone implants for cosmetic reasons do not have this problem. I signed up to be part of the trial with the silicone implants, and am glad to know that a year later the FDA regulated the implants for elective surgery as well. They are safe.

Anyone looking at me as I left the hospital would have easily assumed that I had healthy, well-sized, perfectly normal breasts. They felt and looked perfect to me, but Dr. LaTrenta urged me to consider one more procedure: nipple reconstruction. During my mastectomy, my nipples were not reattached because there was a risk that they may contain cancer cells. For that reason, reattaching a woman's original nipples are never part of

After Surgery: The PT Prescription

Shoulder pain and a loss of strength in the arm are common in many women after breast surgery. A study published in 2007 reported that physical therapy is very effective in easing pain and increasing mobility after breast surgery. Sessions usually include gentle stretching, range of motion exercises and massage. In this particular study the women who received physical therapy showed "significant improvement in shoulder mobility and had significantly less pain than the control group." Before participating in the study, most of the women said that they avoided social activities because of their pain and stiffness. After the three- and six-month trials, the group that received physical therapy said that they enjoyed a significant improvement in their quality of life.

Source: "Physiotherapy Helpful After Breast Cancer Surgery,"

breastcancer.org

breast reconstruction, but nipples can be created from the woman's own skin and attached as the last phase. Both Dr. LaTrenta and Dr. Osborne pushed me to get this done. Doctor LaTrenta felt like the artist who didn't have a chance to finish his painting, but I wasn't sure if I wanted to have this procedure. With two successful surgeries behind me, I felt it would be greedy and vain to go back for more. I was healthy and feeling great. Why rock the boat with another surgery?

For many women nipples are erotic zones, but it was never that way for me. I had always associated nipples with my mother's disease and never derived a special pleasure from them. My breast reconstruction had given me the gift of retaining some sensation in my skin, and I was grateful for that. I enjoy the sensual feeling of my skin, and I didn't think nipples were important enough to mean enduring another surgical procedure. On the other hand, without nipples not a day went by that I wasn't reminded of the fear and pain I had endured by getting my cancer diagnosis and losing my breasts. I felt healthy, but the blank-looking surface of my naked breasts also made me feel like damaged goods. Both of my surgeons were adamant that I would feel much more whole and self-confident after nipple reconstruction. Throughout my cancer experience they had shown nothing but genuine concern and compassion for me, and they had always delivered much more than I dreamed was possible. I trusted them and finally decided to take their advice and have one more procedure.

For me, nipple reconstruction was the most uncomfortable procedure I had in the course of my cancer treatment. About one year after my implant surgery, Dr. LaTrenta harvested skin grafts from the tender skin in my groin area, which left the area very sensitive and painful. I could not wear panties for about two and a half months because they irritated the healing skin, so I was forced to wear loose sweatpants to work. I made the best of it by finding black or gray sweatpants with a matching long blazer, and no one noticed, but the pain was tough.

During minor surgery in his office, Dr. LaTrenta attached a pair of amazingly realistic-looking nipples. When the bandages came off two weeks later and I saw my reflection in the mirror, I knew he'd been right all along. He is truly an artist, and we both deserved to allow him to finish his masterpiece.

Since completing that surgery, I jump out of the shower and pass in front of the mirror every day without giving a thought to what I went through. My reflection no longer carries reminders of my old fears and pain, but simply reminds me that I have a healthy life ahead filled with opportunities to live out all my dreams.

I took responsibility for finding the best surgeons for my needs and expectations, and I will always be grateful to them and their teams for coming into my life. Today, no woman needs to sacrifice her feminine form to cancer.

When I do spring cleaning in my closets, I grab a few pictures out of their boxes and take a quick glance. Looking at the "before" photos that Daisy took prior to my first surgery makes me feel blessed to be alive and to feel great. I hear so many stories, still, about not-so-lucky outcomes that I feel no regrets for losing both breasts, if that is what it took to get me here today. I still laugh when I think about whomever developed the pictures. I just wanted Daisy to shoot images of my chest, but she was a bozo about it and took pictures of my face, too, so God knows what they were thinking when they developed the pictures.

Putting my surgeries in perspective three years later, I now know that the fear of the unknown was worse than the actual road I travelled. The mastectomy was a challenge to my spirit for a time because initially I felt incomplete, even punished. Physically, it crippled me for a few short weeks, but pain medications kept me from feeling any discomfort. In the

The Latest In Breast Reconstruction: The Nipple-Sparing Mastectomy

One of the newest procedures being studied by reconstructive breast surgeons is the nipple-sparing mastectomy, in which the nipple and surrounding areola are cut away and scraped clean of the breast tissue. If a pathologist determines no breast cancer cells were found near the nipple or areola, the two tissues are reattached.

My reconstructive surgeon, Dr. Gregory LaTrenta, explains that this procedure is still in the early stages:

A woman's breast has two major components to the nipple complex the nipple itself and the thick highly elastic and pigmented circle of skin which surrounds it; the areola. Areola-sparing mastectomy reconstruction has only recently become a standard of care for breast reconstruction patients as five year studies have shown that patients who have had this procedure have recurrence rates similar to non-areola sparing mastectomy patients (when tumors are remote from the areola/nipple complex). Nipple sparing surgery is even newer; therefore, long term studies of its safety and efficacy are not yet available and optimal positioning is very difficult. The technique is considered controversial, and needs to be discussed between a patients and her breast surgeon, depending primarily on the location of the patient's tumor and her pathology.

grand scheme of things that radical surgery made me healthy again and probably saved my life.

Tips

- ❖ Many insurance plans include physical therapy, but some require a doctor's referral. Check out your insurance plan carefully before you begin your treatment.

- ❖ Most group insurance plans cover every aspect of breast cancer treatment, including surgery, breast reconstruction and follow-up treatments for issues that may come up after surgery. Most plans also include prescription drug coverage, so talk to your insurance provider about how much of your chemotherapy will be covered. Today, many insurance companies also provide coverage for alternative therapies like acupuncture and massage. Avoid the added stress of worrying about your coverage and talk to your human resources department at work about your coverage as soon as possible. I found that doctors were very cooperative in making payment arrangements for out-of-pocket expenses, so the sooner you can make those arrangements and gain peace of mind, the better.

- ❖ If you do not have insurance, there are many programs available to help. You can find a listing of government and non-profit resources at the National Cancer Institute (www.cancer.gov) and of local and national breast cancer organization resources at www.cancercare.org. In addition, your hospital or cancer center may have a special fund for women who cannot afford care. Speak to the financial or social services department to ask about this.

To make your post-surgery hospital stay as comfortable as possible:

❖ I spoke to some women who only wanted immediate family in the hospital when they woke up. They didn't want any visitors. Don't be a superhero! Reach out for support. I wanted everyone I love to be around me when I woke up in the recovery room, and that's what I got. It was good for everyone. Your family and friends want to be there for you, so lean on them.

❖ I highly recommend bringing your favorite pictures, socks, blanket and pillow to make your room feel more like home.

❖ If you don't have a refrigerator in the room, bring a cooler to keep your favorite waters and beverages close at hand.

❖ Flowers are lovely gifts from visitors, but keep in mind that you will not be able to lift anything for weeks. Ask friends or family to limit flowers or, after you get home, to change the water in the vases for you.

❖ The hospital will provide a "mastectomy bra" for you. Ask your plastic surgeon for a list of shops that carry mastectomy bras, swimsuits and other garments so that you can choose your own items, too. The office managers or nurses in your doctors' offices are a wealth of good information about this and many other post-surgery concerns.

❖ Use this time to work on a schedule for those who are going to help you with your drains after you return home.

Chapter 4

Chemo

"Sickness shows us what we are."

–Latin Proverb

Mention the word chemotherapy to anyone and images of hair loss and nausea come to mind. After my mastectomy, just the thought of my upcoming chemotherapy treatments hit me hard. A few weeks before my first chemo treatment, my friend Anne picked me up to take me to dinner. Before we got to the restaurant she had to pull to the side of the road, and I got violently sick. I cried because I never throw up. "It's the chemo!" I told Anne. She leaned over, grabbed me by the shoulders and said "You haven't started the chemo yet. Stop it!" My anxiety over the unknown was in full swing.

After getting my results back from the mastectomy, Dr. Osborne thought that because the margins around the original tumor were clear of cancer, chemotherapy wasn't absolutely necessary. I endorsed his thinking. I didn't want to have chemotherapy. But the decision was too important to base on my surgeon's recommendation and my reluctance to go through with the treatment, so I made appointments with three oncologists at Cornell to get their opinions.

It was a good move because each of them took many factors into play, which indicated that chemotherapy was necessary. I trusted them with their specialty, just as I trusted my surgeons with theirs.

When choosing an oncologist among the three I met, I considered the fact that I would ultimately see this doctor once a year for the rest of my life. The follow-up would involve blood tests and talking over the results, but the interaction wasn't at the same critical level of surgery. I wanted to work with someone who made me feel comfortable and was well respected in the field. Doctor Ellen Chuang had been recommended to me by Dr. Osborne's office manager, Susan. She told me that although Dr. Chuang was new to the hospital, she was extremely knowledgeable and experienced, and she

Just like in most important areas of life, it takes a village to put together the expertise that cancer treatment requires.

Today's Four Standard Breast Cancer Treatments

I. Surgery

Most patients with breast cancer have surgery to remove the cancer from the breast. Surgery options, as outlined on page 58, range from lumpectomy to total mastectomy. Usually, some of the lymph nodes under the arm are also taken out and examined for cancer cells.

II. Radiation Therapy

This treatment uses high-energy x-rays or other types of radiation to kill cancer cells or keep them from growing. External radiation therapy uses a machine outside the body to send radiation toward the cancer, and the second type, internal radiation, places a sealed radioactive substance directly into or near the cancer. When there is no cancer found in the lymph nodes, as was my case, radiation therapy is not necessary after a mastectomy.

III. Chemotherapy

Chemotherapy uses drugs to stop the growth of cancer cells, either by killing the cells or by stopping them from dividing. When chemotherapy is taken by mouth or injected into a vein or muscle, the drugs enter the bloodstream and can reach cancer cells throughout the body.

IV. Hormone Therapy

Hormone therapy—which I think would better be called "anti-hormone therapy"—removes hormones or blocks their action and stops cancer cells from growing. Some hormones that circulate through our bloodstream can cause certain cancers to grow. Estrogen, for example, makes some breast cancers grow, and hormone therapy that stops the ovaries from making estrogen is called ovarian ablation.

Hormone therapy with tamoxifen is often given to patients with early stages of breast cancer and those with metastatic breast cancer (cancer that has spread to other parts of the body). Hormone therapy with the drug called tamoxifen or estrogens can act on cells all over the body and may increase the chance of developing endometrial cancer. Women taking tamoxifen should have a pelvic exam every year to look for any signs of cancer. Any vaginal bleeding, other than menstrual bleeding, should be reported to a doctor as soon as possible.

Hormone therapy with an aromatase inhibitor is given to some older, postmenopausal women who have hormone-dependent breast cancer, which needs the hormone estrogen to grow. Aromatase inhibitors decrease the body's estrogen by blocking an enzyme called aromatase from turning androgen into estrogen.

Source: National Cancer Institute

knew I would like her. When I met Dr. Chuang, I was surprised by her youthful appearance. She looked like a 20-year-old, not a wife and mother with more than a decade of medical practice under her belt. She was smart, savvy and confident. But I must admit, even more important, she took my insurance. The other two oncologists were also excellent, but I would have had to pay about $5,000 out of pocket for each appointment. That fact clinched my decision, but it didn't mean I had any doubts about Dr. Chuang's expertise.

After choosing Dr. Chuang, my team of physicians was complete. Just like in most important areas of life, it takes a village to put together the expertise that cancer treatment requires. As it turned out, it was helpful to have each of my physicians affiliated with the same hospital because they had easy access to my records and to each other. This streamlined almost every process, but it didn't mean they would agree on everything. All three opinions I received from the oncologists I met with differed from Dr. Osborne's. They looked at my tests from the more specialized view of oncology, and the statistics they pulled together determined that I needed chemotherapy.

In rare cases, some chemotherapy drugs may weaken the heart muscle or cause a heart attack, especially during the IV infusion of the drugs. I was deathly afraid of my heart not being able to endure it. Doctor Chuang was thorough about covering these risks, no matter how small, and for a few days I let my fears get the best of me. I had watched too many Lifetime movies about people battling cancer and going through hell on chemo with vomiting, diarrhea and excruciating pain. How could a person endure it? Those images, on top of memories of my mother's experience and the thought of losing my hair, added up to a lot of anxiety. In truth, however, chemo wasn't nearly as bad as I thought it would be.

During my weeks of chemotherapy I slept a lot, didn't eat much and was extremely fatigued. After coming home from a treatment, I would take a nap and worry about how I would feel when I woke up, but was always pleasantly surprised that it wasn't that bad. Sleepiness made me feel like I lost a day here and there, and minor concerns like heartburn and checking for canker sores were annoying issues that needed attention. But overall, the drugs that Dr. Chuang prescribed to ease the nausea, the efforts I took to keep my immune system strong and the non-stop support I received from my friends and family made chemo a much less traumatic experience than I anticipated.

Dr. Chuang scheduled me for four cycles of chemotherapy, a combination of Adriamycin and Cytoxin, every two weeks. This mix of drugs would attack cancerous cells from different angles. In my case, with early-stage breast cancer, the chemotherapy was required to prevent recurrence. This is known as adjuvant chemotherapy.

I have never been a person to do things half assed so I agreed with Dr. Chuang's protocol and started researching how I could get through the treatments with the fewest side effects. Chemotherapy is given in cycles, one treatment every two weeks, so that you can recover before your next treatment. Because I was young, Dr. Chuang scheduled the treatments quite far apart so that my reproductive system would remain healthy. Some women never get their period back and become infertile after chemotherapy, so it's very important to consider this when faced with a chemo regimen. Having cancer is a major health crisis in and of itself, but facing the loss of one's ability to biologically have children significantly adds to the crisis. The pros and cons were clear: undergoing chemotherapy would reduce the chances of my cancer reappearing, but it would also factor in the new risks of possible heart failure and early menopause. I didn't want to do the chemotherapy, but God forbid the cancer came back. I didn't want to go through it all again.

Doctor Chuang was patient with all my questions and treated me with compassion. I never felt rushed with her, and when I wasn't in her

Facts About Chemo and Fertility

➤ You many experience a temporary loss of your period during chemotherapy. It may return in a few months or as long as a year after your treatment is over.

➤ Your age has a lot to do with whether or not you become infertile after chemotherapy.
The younger you are, the better the chances that your ovaries will continue to produce eggs. Women nearer age 51, the average age of menopause (when the eggs naturally stop producing eggs), have a stronger chance of becoming infertile after chemotherapy.

➤ Age 35 is the boundary at which you become more apt to have permanent ovarian shutdown, and it is even more of a possibility after age 40.

➤ High overall doses of chemo increase your chances of infertility.

➤ Certain types of chemotherapy drugs have a greater chance of damaging the ovaries than others. Common chemo drugs and their affect on infertility are:

High risk: Cytoxan (cyclophosphamide)
Medium risk: Platinol (cisplatin) and Adriamycin (doxorubicin)
Little or no risk: Amethopterin (methotrexate), Adrucil (5-fluorouracil,
fluorouracil or 5-FU), and Oncovin (vincristine)

➤ The odds vary greatly among individual women, but on average, about 50 percent of women under age 35 resume their period after chemotherapy.

➤ A fertility counselor can guide you through your specific risk and recommend options like egg harvesting prior to chemo. You may produce fewer eggs after chemo, so other fertility options may be necessary.

➤ Your body needs at least sixth months to recover from chemo so that eggs that were damaged can repair themselves. Your doctor will advise that you wait at least that long to try to get pregnant.

Source: Breastcancer.org

office she was always an email away. I admire her patience to this day because I wasn't a model patient by any means. The first month, while we made preparations for starting the chemo treatments, I learned that I couldn't eat sweets during chemo so I ate all my favorites—a lot. I ate like I was going to the electric chair and she wasn't pleased. She kindly but firmly encouraged me to eat better, but I went overboard and gained 10 pounds.

Our appointments dealt with much more than chemotherapy. Doctor Chuang always emphasized lifestyle choices that would lower the chances of the cancer returning, such as minimal alcohol consumption and no smoking. I wasn't a big drinker or a smoker, so I knew those rules would be easy to follow. To keep me as healthy as possible during chemo, she recommended that I do any kind of regular exercise, drink a lot of fluids and wash my hands constantly to avoid infections. At every appointment I asked the same questions about the chances of the cancer returning, my life expectancy, how long it would take my hair to grow back and how much my fertility would be affected.

Some women choose to have an egg-harvesting procedure before chemotherapy so that they have an option for in vitro fertilization if the chemo does too much harm to their ovaries. Doctor Chuang gave me this option, but also explained that she didn't think my fertility would be in jeopardy because of my young age and the two-week breaks between the chemo sessions, which would be less intense on my system than sessions placed more closely together.

Week after week, Dr. Chuang had her hands full with me. When she recommended a cream to prevent canker sores that was not specifically indicated for that condition, I had a hard time being convinced that it was okay. I was used to reading all the fine print that comes in drug packaging, so when Dr. Chuang told me to put the cream in my mouth at the first sign of irritation, but the label stated "do not ingest," I called her several times to make sure I understood her orders. I should have trusted her in the first place because she was right on the money, it really worked. The cream made my tiny canker sores disappear immediately and they never developed into real sores.

I also took time at our appointments to tell her about the alternative approaches I had heard about and taken up, such as taking vitamins and drinking a lot of green tea and pomegranate juice. She listened, but she wasn't a big proponent of these things. She told me that I could continue what I was doing because it wouldn't hurt me, but she made it clear that she didn't consider it real medicine.

Suggested Easy-On-the-Stomach Foods

Meals & Snacks

Chicken - broiled or baked, without the skin

Cream of Wheat® or Cream of Rice® cereal

Crackers or pretzels

Oatmeal

Pasta or noodles

Potatoes - boiled, without the skin

White rice

Soups

Clear broth, such as chicken, beef, and vegetable

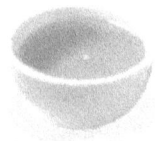

Fruits & Sweets

Bananas

Canned fruit such as applesauce, peaches, and pears

Gelatin (Jell-O®)

Popsicles and sherbet

Yogurt (plain or vanilla)

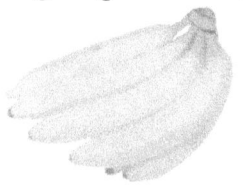

Drinks

Clear soda such as:
 ginger ale
Cranberry or grape juice

Oral rehydration solution drinks, such as:
Pedialyte®

Tea, Water

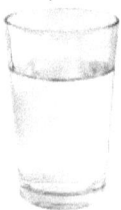

Source: National Cancer Institute

When I asked her if I could expect to live for five, ten or twenty years, I always expected a tough answer. It was a terrible concern, so I kept asking. I couldn't let go of it. She wouldn't promise me anything, no one could, but she always told me I'd be okay. With my early diagnosis, no lymph involvement, young age, healthy lifestyle and phenomenal job Drs. Osborne and LaTrenta had done on my surgeries, she was extremely positive about my potential for living a long life. Her confidence always put me at ease.

Each appointment began with Dr. Chuang examining my chest to see how well it was healing and to make sure there was no infection around the tubes to my tissue expanders. Then we would talk about my concerns and discuss the progress of my chemotherapy course. With all three doctors in the same hospital, my appointments went very smoothly. My schedule started with Dr. Osborne for a quick examination of the surgical healing, then I visited Dr. LaTrenta for another tissue expander exam. Next I went to Dr. Chuang's office on the same floor, and after that appointment walked across the hall to the lab for blood work. Making all these rounds on one day limited my travel time, which helped me get a lot of rest the rest of the week. I followed every word of their advice and forced myself to eat healthy food, take regular walks in the park, allow my support system to take care of me and keep a positive attitude. With all that ammunition, my cancer didn't have a chance.

I needed to be brave and hit the cancer with everything I had. Not everyone agreed with my decision, which became a much bigger issue than I ever imagined it would be. My father desperately tried to talk me out of doing it. He was haunted by the vivid memory of how chemotherapy destroyed his beautiful wife and, after all that suffering, didn't even cure her. He recalled the vomiting and the pain and he wanted to protect me from that. When I stood my ground, he talked to my friends and asked them to try to change my mind.

Another person who disagreed with my choice was my long-time friend Denise. We were like sisters and I couldn't imagine my life without her. Our families were very close, and when Denise's Mom died of

Infection Risk: Your white blood cell count (WBC) will go low about 10-14 days after each chemotherapy treatment and will take a few days to go back to normal. To lower your risk for infections, try to avoid crowds or people with the flu or colds. Wash uncooked fruits and vegetables before eating. If you have a temperature of 100.5 or higher, shaking, chills, a productive cough, burning with urination or other signs/symptoms of infection, call your doctor.

stomach cancer two years earlier, I took time off work to attend the wake and funeral and distract the young kids in the family with treats. When I got my breast cancer diagnosis, I needed Denise. I had no idea that she would be so opposed to my decision to have chemotherapy. She saw how it destroyed her mother and she, like my Dad, wanted to spare me the emotional and physical pain. I explained that her Mom's side effects were more severe than mine would be because her Mom's body was already stressed out from drinking and smoking, which she didn't give up during chemotherapy. But nothing I said could win her support. I called her after every round to let her know I was okay, but she never called back. There was no doubt that Denise loved me and couldn't bear to lose me. She was with Ivette when I woke up from surgery, bawling her eyes out with happiness. Ivette later told me that Denise had been a train wreck the entire time I was in surgery. But her emotional response to her mother's death was too powerful to keep us together.

Chemotherapy was my insurance plan, and a lot of my anxiety gave way to a sense of hope and security. At the same time, I knew that it wasn't going to be a joy ride. In order to kill the bad cells, the medicine damages healthy cells and organs as well, which creates unpleasant side effects. The prospect of chemotherapy was certainly frightening, but understanding how it worked alleviated some of my fears.

In one of my pre-chemo appointments with Dr. Chuang, she filled me in on the sophisticated new drugs that help alleviate some of the common side effects. When she described how anti-nausea medications like Anzemat, Zofran and Kytril work, all I could think of was how different my mother's fight with cancer would have been if such drugs had been available—not to speak of the more powerful cancer-killing drugs themselves. The nausea-reducing drugs are taken on the evening of a chemo session and over the next three days. A milder drug called Compazine takes care of low-level nausea, and Ativan (lorazepam) tackles both nausea and anxiety. I was grateful for this double-duty medication because it took the edge off my anxiety and worked very well on the nausea.

I showed up at the eighth floor of the Cornell Medical Building once every two weeks for my treatments, and in the process discovered an entire subculture of women who were going through their own battles. The room, which was always freezing cold, reminded me of a nail salon with its six large, pedicure-type chairs. I once asked Dr. Chuang why the room was so cold, thinking that maybe the medicines needed to stay cool. She

Why the Nausea?

Nausea—the feeling that you are going to throw up—and vomiting itself are common side effects of chemotherapy.

Chemotherapy drugs cause these side effects by sending chemical messages to parts of the brain and spinal cord that regulate nausea and vomiting. Some messages go to the Chemoreceptor Trigger Zone (CTZ) an area of the brain that sends signals to the brain's vomiting center. The drugs also do some damage to stomach cells, which causes the release of a neurotransmitter called serotonin. This neurotransmitter sends a signal about the damaged to the brain's vomiting center.

Your doctor can recommend a variety of prescription medicines that can combat both. You may need to go through a process of trial and error to find the one that works best for you.

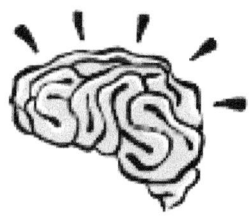

laughed and said no; it was probably just poor engineering in the building! Each woman usually came with a friend or relative or two who sat in regular chairs and visited while the medicine dripped into our veins through the IVs. There were never more than three of us receiving chemo at the same time, and the atmosphere was unlike any other place I've ever been. Combined with the patient and compassionate attitude of our nurse, Nicole, was the love and support flowing from the visitors who had come with us. Along with the strangeness of the tubes and the big chairs, the seriousness of the situation and the weird smell—I never figured out where it came from—there was a lot of love in that room.

We exchanged ideas, shared tips about strengthening our immune systems, and reassured and comforted each other. We learned about someone's favorite over-the-counter product for constipation, a common side effect, and the fantastic alcohol-free mouthwashes that saved some of us from getting canker sores. We talked about how important it was to avoid crowds and wash our uncooked fruits and vegetables to keep the germs at bay while our systems were so weakened. We asked Nicole if she had learned of any new anti-nausea or anti-anxiety medications that had just come on the market, and we shared our methods for relaxing and keeping our minds busy on something other than cancer: like surfing the Internet and actually *doing* the crafts that Martha

Nausea-reducing drugs are taken on the evening of a chemo session and over the next three days. A milder drug called Compazine takes care of low-level nausea, and Ativan (lorazepam) tackles both nausea and anxiety.

Stewart occupies herself with on TV.

I will never forget one woman, God Bless her, who rocked my boat. We asked her what sort of chemo treatment she was receiving, and she said "Three," which I thought meant a mix of three medicines. I said, "Me, too," but then she explained that it was her third chemo cocktail, her third go-round, because her cancer had metastasized. The room went silent. What a brave and gutsy woman. It made my problems seem small.

So many of my friends came along to my treatments over the course of those months. We never forgot why we were there, of course, so there was always trepidation walking in and walking out, and a few tears. But soon we would lose ourselves in normal talk about Mio's son Joaquin, Anne's beautiful new house, or where we were going for lunch afterward. The familiar conversation was like a warm blanket that protected me from fear and loncliness as I put my body through hell. My friends knew that it was enough to just be with me and talk about real life, the small things that make life worth living. I'm forever grateful.

We always went to lunch after chemo because on days three through seven after a treatment I couldn't eat. My nausea was too severe. It was bad, even with the anti-nausea drugs, so I couldn't imagine what my mother's nausea had been like. Ironically, I loved watching the Food

Network on those days. I can truly say Bobby Flay, Rachel Ray and all those great chefs lifted my spirits tremendously. I wrote down all the recipes and as nauseous as I was, I cooked elaborate meals for my brother and my friends. I had never been interested in cooking shows before, but I became hooked and watched them about ten hours a day. So, oddly enough, I can thank chemotherapy for making me a really great cook.

I stocked the house with cases of water, movies, medications and toiletries. Frozen fruit pops and boiled apples with cinnamon were my favorite foods on my bad days. Baked potatoes, soda crackers and gelatin desserts also curbed the nausea and tasted great. Chinese green tea was very soothing as well.

My friends were careful not to come around if they felt sick because the chemo compromised my immune system and I was hyper-vulnerable to infection. I also got nauseous if my bladder was full, so I went to the bathroom a lot after a chemo sessions. Usually I could hold on until I found a super clean restroom (that's the germophobe in me), but while I was on

Healing Dry Skin During Chemo: I used Vaseline to reduce dryness on my face and hands. It works great and is inexpensive. I also swore by Shisheido Bio Performance, which I applied morning and night. It's expensive, but it really kept my skin hydrated.

chemotherapy I didn't have that luxury. It was a crazy side effect that I didn't expect.

By the time I felt I was getting back to normal, it was time to return to the room with the big chairs and blast myself with poison again. The drugs faded my tan and gave me white, pale glow, which a lot of my friends thought looked great. Friends and strangers would stop and ask me what my beauty regimen was, and I replied "chemo." We always got a chuckle out of that. Before my first chemo treatment I was a size 4 and weighed 130 pounds. After chemo I was down to 110, and I actually looked better. Those positive side effects didn't quite make up for the harshness of chemotherapy, however. The third session was particularly rough. It was like going sailing and expecting the tides to be one to two feet, when if fact they are a powerful six to eight feet. Like the other women I met during treatments, I coped and continued to count down the days to my final session.

My favorite uncles from Argentina, Claudio and Alfredo, came to New York to celebrate my upcoming last chemo treatment. They had no idea what to expect, but would not have been surprised to find a bedridden niece. I got as pretty as I could and went out with them several times. I

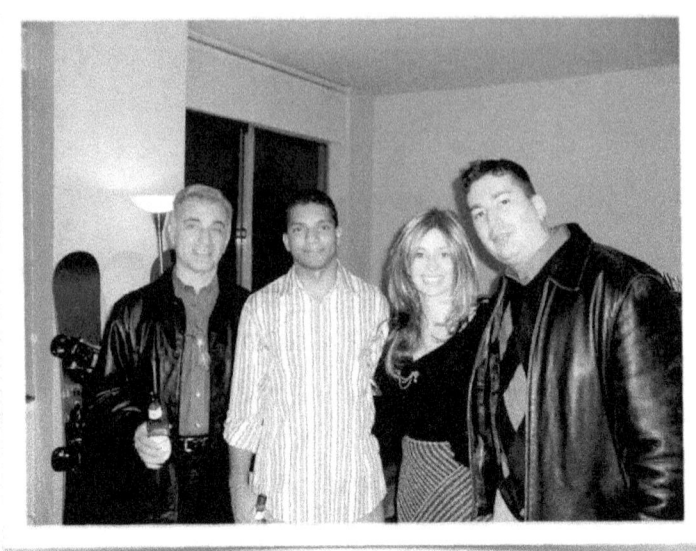

Uncle Claudio, my friend Sachin, me (in a quirky wig) and my brother, Josi

was still weak from the surgeries and treatments, but it was worth it to push myself and let them cheer me on.

I think my uncles thought they made the trip to say goodbye to me. When they saw my zest for life and how well I maintained myself, they were pleasantly surprised. Josi took them sightseeing a few hours every day while I stayed home and slept, and in the evenings we stayed home or went out to eat. I sensed that they were uncomfortable about asking for details of my treatment,so we didn't talk about the nitty gritty very much. They were grateful when I volunteered information, but they didn't ask too many questions. I made sure to tell them about my chances of having children after chemotherapy because I knew this was a concern among the entire family. I let them know that my odds were very good. Overall, they couldn't believe the difference in my condition compared to what they remembered of my mother's experience with breast cancer. Uncle Claudio said that on a scale of 1 to 10, 1 being bad 10 being terrible, my Mom's cancer had been a 12 and a 5 for me.

Most of my life before, during and after breast cancer has revolved around food, and by the time my uncles came to visit I was nearing the end of chemo and could eat my own cooking. I fixed huge breakfasts and, when I wanted to get out of the kitchen, took them to some of New York's best traditional places like Junior's Cheesecake in Brooklyn. There are only one or two types of cheesecake made in Argentina, so when we went to Junior's I ordered 20 different kinds and we had a party. They were overwhelmed.

One night we went to a Halloween party and I was uncomfortable because I was still bald and didn't know what to wear for a costume. I had lost about 20 pounds since starting chemo, so I went to my closet and found the skinniest pieces I owned, leather pants and cute pink top. To top it off I put on the short, bright pink wig Josi had bought me just for fun, and it looked

My Tools

Positive Thinking
Knowledge
Self-empowerment

adorable. Josi and my uncles dressed in the scrubs I got from the hospital, and we got to the party I felt very comfortable. My coloring was getting better and I felt like I fit in. It was my real first outing and I felt like the old me. My uncles were delighted to see me happy and dancing up a storm.

After my uncles left, I faced my final round of chemo. The third round had been hard, but the last one wiped me out. Two weeks afterward I began throwing up four times a day and ran a fever. I thought I could shake it off at home, but I became so sick that I moved into my Dad's house so that he and Josi could take care of me. This crushed my ego because I had never had to depend on them to that extent. I felt more sick than I had ever felt from the effects of chemo. The pain was horrific and left me bedridden. I was so weak that I couldn't even get up to move my car for alternative parking, so my friend Irene did it for me. I lay in the guest room bed at Dad's house dizzy with fever and horrible headaches, sweating profusely, vomiting and feeling cramps so severe that I expected to find a baby at the end of the bed. A few days after moving to Dad's, my friend Anne visited me and forced me to go to the hospital, thank God. After I was admitted, my fever got worse, rising to 106.5 degrees, and I learned that I was passing kidney stones and suffering from a kidney

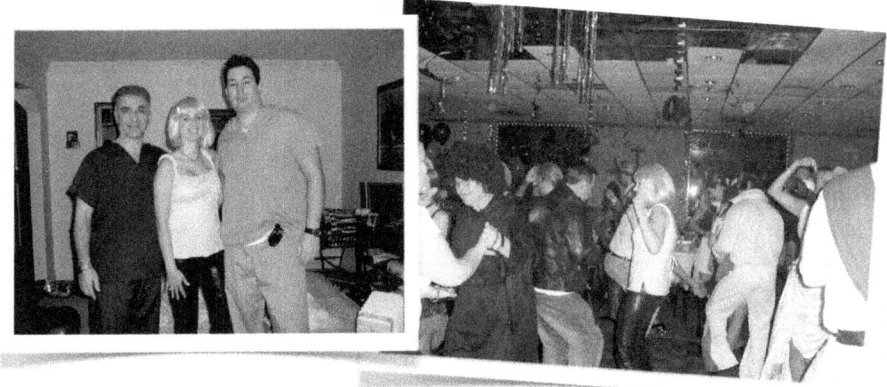

Ready for Halloween in my pink wig.

infection. Lying bedridden in the hospital for nearly a week wouldn't be fun, but it could have been a lot worse.

Two IVs filled with antibiotics prevented me from moving my arms for five days, and the constriction was almost unbearable. I fell into a bit of a depressive state." Are you kidding me? "I thought to myself." I had just beaten the chemo and paid my dues. But no, I have to deal with kidney stones and a kidney infection, too? "

I brought the kidney infection largely on myself because I had not been drinking enough fluids and was severely dehydrated. Doctor Chuang ordered me to drink 8 to 10 bottles of water a day, but even drinking a half glass felt like too much. I always felt so full, like I couldn't swallow a drop, and I didn't force myself to drink like I should have. On good days I was the perfect patient, but on bad days I was stubborn and just wanted to be left alone.

A Glimpse at Tomorrow's Breast Cancer Treatments

Several new treatments that are now being tested in clinical trials include:

Sentinel Lymph Node Biopsy

This method allows surgeons to remove fewer lymph glands during breast cancer surgery. At the beginning of surgery, a radioactive substance or dye is injected near the tumor. The liquid flows through the lymph ducts to the lymph nodes, and the surgeon removes the first lymph node that receives the substance. This tissue is sent to a lab, where it is examined for cancer cells. If no cells are present, the odds are good that cancer has not spread to any other tissues and it may not be necessary to remove any more lymph nodes. After this procedure, the surgeon completes the breast surgery.

High-dose Chemotherapy with Stem Cell Transplant

This treatment uses high doses of chemotherapy and replaces blood-forming cells that were destroyed by the cancer treatment. Stem cells (immature blood cells) are removed from the blood or bone marrow of the patient or a donor and are frozen and stored. After the chemotherapy is completed, the stored stem cells are thawed and given back to the patient through an infusion. These reinfused stem cells grow into (and restore) the body's blood cells. So far, studies have shown that this treatment does not work better than standard chemotherapy, so it will be some time before it is introduced beyond clinical trials.

Monoclonal Antibodies as Adjuvant Therapy

Antibodies made in the laboratory from a single type of immune system cell are used in this treatment. These antibodies can identify substances on cancer cells that may help cancer cells grow. The antibodies attach to the substances and kill the cancer cells, block their growth, or keep them from spreading. (Adjuvant therapies are treatments given after the main treatment, surgery, to help prevent recurrence.)

Tyrosine Kinase Inhibitors as Adjuvant Therapy

Tyrosine kinase inhibitors are drugs that block signals needed for tumors to grow.

Source: National Cancer Institute

The infectious disease specialist who treated me had to experiment with various antibiotics because treating someone who is undergoing chemotherapy (or recently had her last treatment, like I had) requires special measures. He was concerned that my immune system may not be strong enough to let the drugs work, so he put me on a broad spectrum of antibiotics. He told me that if the drugs kicked in, I would be fine. And fortunately, they did.

My fuel tank felt empty after just a few hours lying in the hospital, but I quickly learned that I had more on reserve. With the help of a great doctor, nursing staff and my support system, I drummed up enough patience and strength to hang in and get past it. My friend Michael Uhrin makes fun of me now when he remembers my first day in the hospital when he and my dear friend, Leslie, visited. I wanted nothing to eat from the outside. But by day four I was giving them a $50 lunch order. Lobster this, mozzarella that, cobb salad, and don't forget dessert—surprise me. I was feeling more like myself.

Throughout my weeks of cancer treatment, I gradually learned to rely on others and let my friends and relatives take care of me. I had always been very active and independent, cramming twenty projects into a day. Just resting and letting others help me was very humbling. My friend Irene came over almost every day like a "drive by" to see if I needed any errands done. In spite of how much I stocked up on food and supplies (so no one would have to shop for me and I'd feel like I was still in control), every once in awhile I needed more fruit or water or crackers, and she made sure I had them. Leaning on friends may take some getting used to, but it's an important part of healing.

I gained things from chemo that went far beyond destroying the cancer. I gained assurance. I also lost a few things like my hair and my friendship with Denise. The following year she called and apologized for not being there for me. I told her I forgave her and loved her. I said that I was feeling great, back to work and living in a house I had bought in Queens. We've seen each other twice since then, but it's not the same as it was before. It's still strange to realize that I lost a good friend to choosing a treatment to save my life.

There were times I wanted to quit chemotherapy, especially when everyone was going to the beach and soaking up the sun. But I made myself step back and look at the big picture. I could easily let go of one summer if it meant fifty more summers at the beach. Most of all, I wanted to grow old with my family and friends.

Here are more tips I learned from health professionals and my fellow chemotherapy patients that helped me during my treatment:

❖ For constipation, over-the-counter products like Correctol, Colace, Milk of Magnesia and Senonkot are helpful. Drinking lots of fluids and eating high fiber foods like vegetables, bran, apples, prunes, raisins and apricots are also advised.

❖ Mouth care: the gums, tongue and teeth may be more sensitive while on chemotherapy, and the drugs can cause mouth sores. Think ahead and schedule a teeth cleaning prior to starting chemotherapy so that you can take care of small problems before they begin, and avoid the need for dental work while you're in chemo treatment.

❖ I highly recommend products like Biotene mouthwash and toothpaste to boost your mouth's defense system and prevent mouth discomfort. I never got mouth sores while I was on chemo because I obsessed about these products. They don't taste wonderful, but they're worth it. I met women at chemo treatments with ten or more painful sores in their mouths. Avoid alcohol-containing mouthwashes like Listerine because they can be irritating.

❖ Try to avoid having any dental work during chemo unless absolutely necessary. If you must have dental work done, have your blood count checked beforehand, as the chemo may have lowered your white blood cell count. A low white blood cell count, also called neutropenia, makes it more difficult for you to fight off infection, so dental work is risky while you're in that condition.

❖ Do not take aspirin or Tylenol to lower fever 10-14 days after chemo, especially when counts are at their lowest. Your doctor needs to know if you are running a fever so that your white blood cell count can be watched carefully.

❖ Reducing Nausea: It is helpful to chew your food thoroughly and relax during meals. Eat small meals often and do not eat 3 to 4 hours before treatment. Take the extra burden off your system by learning stress reduction exercises. Ask your oncologist and nurses about any new drugs that have come on the market to reduce nausea and vomiting.

❖ Make copies of the following page and use the sheet to record your chemotherapy side effects so that you can discuss them with your oncologist.

Keeping Track of Chemotherapy Side Effects

Here's a form to help you keep track of eating-related side effects you may experience while you are undergoing cancer treatment. You can share it with the health professional who is keeping track of side effects with you during this time.

Your name: _____

Week of: _____

Write the type and date of your last treatments(s):

Type of treatment: _____ **Date:** _____

Type of treatment: _____ **Date:** _____

Your Weight: _____ **lbs.** (measure once a week)

Below you will find a list of some eating-related side effects that cancer patients may experience. Check the box next to any side effect listed below that you experience in the week you have listed above. Next to each one you have checked, write a number from 1 to 3 indicating how severe you think each side effect was for you, where:

1= mild; 2= moderate; and 3= severe.

Side Effect	M	T	W	T	F	S	Sun
Sore/ Dry Mouth	___	___	___	___	___	___	___
Nausea	___	___	___	___	___	___	___
Vomiting	___	___	___	___	___	___	___
Diarrhea	___	___	___	___	___	___	___
Fatigue	___	___	___	___	___	___	___
Other:_____	___	___	___	___	___	___	___

Source: National Cancer Institute

Other Questions or Concerns (Use this space to write down questions or concerns you may want to talk about with your health care provider.)

Chapter 5

WHEN DEPRESSION IS NOT A DIRTY WORD

"Let your tears come. Let them water your soul."

—Eileen Mayhew

Before I had cancer I would call in sick at work if I had a pimple on my face because it upset me and made me feel ugly. If Michael and I had a fight I would shut down and stay home. When I didn't get my way at a meeting or was refused something I wanted I would get all stressed out. I wasn't a drama girl every day. Just every now and then I got a little depressed. No matter how good my overall situation was, if something didn't go my way I would make an issue out of it. I have always been very emotional—that's the Taurus in me. I'm stubborn and I admit I've had my share of temper tantrums.

After being diagnosed with breast cancer, I finally had good reason to be depressed. I am human, after all. What else would anyone expect?

The tears were inevitable, but I grieved, endured and moved on. Throughout the process I experienced a new set of feelings and challenges.

I may have let everyday problems get me down once in awhile, but I never took anything or anyone in my life for granted. My Mom dying at the age of 42 taught me that lesson. At an early age, I knew that any of us could lose someone we love in the blink of an eye. This has made me humble and grateful for my terrific family, friends and career. I often pampered myself and my loved ones.

But when I learned I had cancer I couldn't help but think that it wasn't fair. All of a sudden, my "real" life, for which I was so grateful, had to be put on hold. I had taken good care of myself and had a great outlook on life. Tragic things aren't supposed to happen to nice, positive people like me, I thought. The frustration and shock of the diagnosis turned into sadness when I thought about everything that was at stake. What if I didn't make it? A huge sense of loss began building up inside me.

Give Yourself Permission to Grieve

It is normal to feel depressed after receiving bad news like a cancer diagnosis, and it is also important to be honest about your feelings. I needed to give myself permission to feel sad, angry and confused, and also

116

to grieve over what I thought I may have lost. Even with the knowledge that my mother had died young, it still seemed unbelievable that I could face the same thing. I was depressed about the uncertain future of my body. Would I be deformed? Would I lose my feeling of femininity? Would I ever meet a man who didn't mind that I was a cancer survivor (God willing) and had undergone breast surgery? If I survived, would I be able to have children? Would the cancer come back?

There was a lot to feel sad about. I needed to grieve, and fortunately I felt comfortable enough with my friends to cry around them. It is very important to express sadness and grief when it comes up after a crisis like a breast cancer diagnosis. Letting it out by having a good cry for a day or two—or a few, if that's what you need—is healthier than swallowing your tears. Pour it all out so that you can complete that process and move on.

Surrounded by my friends, I felt free to cry and talk about my fears. This is one of the greatest gifts they gave me, because it was the first step in my healing. It is crucial to find at least one person with whom you can express your emotions and talk about everything that is going through your mind after you receive a diagnosis of breast cancer.

When Sadness Is Normal: Take Time to Grieve and Share Your Feelings with Others
Advice from the Lance Armstrong Foundation

Grief can be painful, but it is a normal process that can help you cope with losses and changes that have come into your life as a result of cancer. Important losses that not grieved are difficult to resolve. They can rob you of energy and joy and prevent you from moving forward into a full and productive life. Sometimes survivors come to understand their grief on their own. However, talking with others can help you:

- Recognize your losses
- Express your feelings
- Understand your feelings and reactions as normal
- Find ways to cope
- Feel stronger and more capable than before

Source: www.livestrong.com

It took awhile to get over the shock and sadness, but once I did, I was free to move on and start making a game plan for my recovery. I learned to combat depression by letting myself grieve after my initial diagnosis. Surrounding myself with a strong and loving support system, taking the big decisions about treatment into my own hands, keeping a positive attitude and accepting the fact that this tough part of my life was just as "real" as the rest.

Relationships and Breast Cancer

One of the toughest challenges that came up during my treatment was the impact cancer had on my relationship with Michael. Unfortunately, I became too dependent on him and he wasn't there as much as I needed him. It hurt to know that I didn't come first in his life, and when the hurt came more often than the consoling, I decided to break up with him. It was terribly hard to do because I loved him so much, but I didn't need the additional stress with everything else going on. At first I thought that I should wait until I was completely out of the woods before springing the news on him, just in case I didn't make it. But I loved him too much to do that. It was time to stop hoping that he would get his act together and after six years we would really be a couple. Facing cancer and going through chemotherapy brought me a lot of clarity. I admitted to myself that it

After Your Diagnosis, Lift Your Spirits By:

▸ *Surrounding yourself with what you love, including your friends, family, pets, favorite music and keepsakes*

▸ *Making your home your refuge: pamper yourself in comfort and security*

▸ *Thinking positive and envisioning the best outcomes*

▸ *Knowing that you are a lot stronger and better than breast cancer*

▸ *Accepting the wisdom that every experience helps you grow* wasn't going to happen, and just before my final chemo session I made the decision to break up with Michael for good.

We had split up several times over the years, but we always got back together. I had a high tolerance for putting up with things because when I was a child I got used to making sure everyone else was taken care of. I was not accustomed to putting myself first, but when I got sick I had to make life-or-death choices for myself. Michael and I loved each other a lot, but we were like oil and vinegar. Somebody always had to give in, and it was usually me. We knew the good, the bad and the ugly about each other, so I always wanted to fix things rather than give up on the relationship. Besides, he was a great guy, handsome, very charismatic and we had a wonderful chemistry (most of the time). But after I began fighting cancer, I took a more honest look at him. He didn't invest 100 percent of himself in the relationship, and he probably never would. I needed to move on and invest 100 percent in myself, so I made the decision to split up and stopped taking his phone calls for some time. He kept calling my best friend, trying to find out what he could do to get me back. He said he wanted to get engaged and promised everything would change, but my mind was made up.

With a major breakup on my hands on top of fighting breast cancer, I had plenty of reasons to be depressed. Michael and I fell into the camp of those relationships that are at a high risk of breaking down during a crisis like breast cancer because they were already having problems before the diagnosis. The added stress is just too much, and in my case I believe that cancer sped up a breakup that was destined to happen anyway. The majority of relationships, however, survive the traumatic experience.

According to one study, more than 40 percent of the couples interviewed actually stated that the cancer experience made their relationship stronger! That's great news for men and women who are facing a breast cancer diagnosis. If the foundation of love and compassion is already in place, there is an excellent chance that the couple can grow closer through the journey of healing.

Not all marriages or close relationships survive a breast cancer diagnosis, but research shows that more than half of them do. One study showing that many marriages actually thrive during the experience confirms my belief that breast cancer, like any crisis, can have a positive side.

Oddly enough, Michael and I managed to stay friends after our breakup, and it's been great. We don't argue anymore. We know each other so well that we can listen, give advice and be there for each other.

Every year he helps me put up my Christmas tree. Most people break up

with their boyfriends and that's it, but Michael is still in my life—in a

different way—and still has a little piece of my heart.

Relationships and Breast Cancer: The Numbers Are On Your Side!

✓The majority of marriages remain intact after breast cancer

✓Most marriages that break up after a breast cancer diagnosis are due to problems that were already in place before the diagnosis

✓COMMUNIATION is the key to keeping a marriage healthy during the trauma of breast cancer: couples need to put their feelings into words and talk about the scary issues like potential cancer recurrence, the woman's changing sense of identity, sexuality and intimacy

✓Couples who have survived other life traumas together have more coping skills to work with after a breast cancer diagnosis

✓In one study, "42 percent of the 282 couples interviewed said that the breast cancer experience brought them closer."

Source: "Nurturing Your Relationship After Breast Cancer,"

www.networkofstrength.org

Making the decision to break up with Michael showed me that I

was capable of putting myself first. I had been through other challenges before breast cancer, but none of them had given me as sharp a focus on my here-and-now needs. The car accident taught me that I didn't have to take doctors' prognoses as gospel. After being told I would, at the very least, walk with a limp the rest of my life, I turned my recovery into a mission to prove them wrong and healed perfectly. And that was not the first painful challenge of my adult life.

Many years earlier I had gone through a heartbreaking divorce. My ex-husband was a wonderful guy, but when I married him I wasn't aware that he suffered from a mental illness. I stuck by him for nearly two years because I took my vows seriously. Once I learned about his illness, I wasn't ashamed of it, as many people are, because I worked in the pharmaceutical industry and knew that it was an ailment that could be treated with medication. My ex-husband, however, who had been diagnosed with the illness ten years before he met me, didn't want to take the medication because it made him gain weight. He made a choice that was very difficult for both of us to live with. I knew he was a great person, but that isn't enough for a marriage. He thought people were out to get him, and for a long time I tried to protect him. But when he continued to refuse to take the medication that would give him a normal life, I had to accept the fact that I could not help him. I was 27 years old and the first person I knew to get divorced. That became a double whammy when I became the first person among my friends to get a life-threatening disease.

Nurture Yourself

Soon after learning that I had cancer I reached out for ways to cope and get on a positive track. I realized that I had many great people in my corner who loved me and were not ready to lose me, and I allowed myself to lean on them. My friends were amazing to me. A little love is like a drop of water, and everything my friends did to help me through my fight with cancer came together like a stream to keep me hopeful and refreshed. Little things meant so much, like the friend who picked up a very strong sun block for me in Canada that wasn't available in the U.S. The chemo made me very sensitive to sunlight, and without his thoughtful gift I would not have been able to get out in the sun. Another friend slipped vitamins in my food and beverages when it was too difficult

"Massage is extremely effective in treating post-surgical problems. It can alleviate swelling and pain. Massage also is a general tonic, in that it relaxes people. And with relaxation, people just deal with their stresses better, and their bodies heal better with just about every illness. Massage is also a form of touch therapy, and touch in itself is healing."

—Dan Benor, M.D.

for me to swallow pills. He did this secretly because he knew I was too sensitive to talk about some of the problems that went with chemo. Another friend helped me plan activities for the months ahead to make sure I had exciting events to look forward to. She was one of my cheerleaders, reminding me that there were "only two chemos to go" or "only a few weeks until my hair started to grow out."

Depression and Fatigue

At least 70 percent of cancer patients undergoing chemotherapy suffer from fatigue. Studies have found that although both depression and fatigue are often experienced at the same time during cancer treatment, they are caused by different factors.

So, if your spirits have lifted and you are keeping positive through your treatment, do not be surprised if you remain very tired. The fatigue may be caused by the cancer itself, chemotherapy, anemia, lack of sleep, poor nutrition, hormonal changes or other factors. It is not necessarily a signal of depression.

Self-Care for Fatigue

- Get into the routine of walking or doing some other form of light exercise
- Take short naps throughout the day
- Drink plenty of fluids, but limit or avoid coffee and alcohol
- Eat nutritious food
- Keep track of the time of day when you have the most energy and schedule your main activities for that time to conserve your energy

Sources: American Cancer Institute and Mayo Clinic

Two Recommended Feel-Good Therapies

Therapeutic Massage

Receiving massage therapy after surgery is almost standard practice in Europe and South America, but it hasn't caught on in the United States yet. I hope that it does soon. I had been going to a massage therapist regularly before I was diagnosed with breast cancer, and I continued the sessions throughout my cancer treatment and surgeries. The benefits of therapeutic massage after breast surgery include its ability to help the tissue heal and to prevent blood from clotting around the breast area. Massage also diminishes stress levels through the relaxing effect of the treatment itself and the comfort of talking to a health practitioner whom you come to know and trust. Massage and touch also enhance the immune system, which is an important benefit after any type of surgery. In addition to all those advantages, I found that message therapy helped my breast implants settle in more naturally after my reconstructive surgery. It also helped me feel connected to my entire body, which was very healing. Many insurance plans now cover massage therapy.

Cupping

This 3,000-year-old therapy is believed to help remove toxins from the body, and I found very helpful while undergoing chemotherapy. The practitioner places hot cups on the back that create a vacuum against the skin and encourage blood and lymph flow. The gentle heat feels wonderful. The skin may look a little red afterward, but the treatment is not painful. Gwyneth Paltrow made headlines with cupping a few years ago when she showed up at a film premier in a backless dress that exposed a series of round, red cupping marks on her back. Cupping is offered at many health spas.

For those who do not have a close-knit group of friends and/or family to turn to, or who want to supplement their home-grown support with a group of women who are going through the same ordeal, a breast cancer support group can fill those roles.

The Young Survival Coalition, a group specifically geared to young women with breast cancer, helped me make decisions and provided a lot of emotional support, enthusiasm and encouragement. Because fewer young women get breast cancer than post-menopausal women, many of them do not have contact with women their age who are going through the same experience. The YSC was set up to meet that special need, with opportunities for women to network, resources for learning about treatment options and much more (youngsurvival.org). I was fortunate to have friends my own age to talk to, as well as two women at work who were in various stages of the disease, but the YSC was an important addition to my network of support.

Another great way to connect with other women who have been diagnosed with breast cancer is to join online chat sessions and support groups, which are available on websites such as Susan G. Komen for the Cure, American

There are more than 250,000 women age 40 and under in the U.S. living with breast cancer.

127

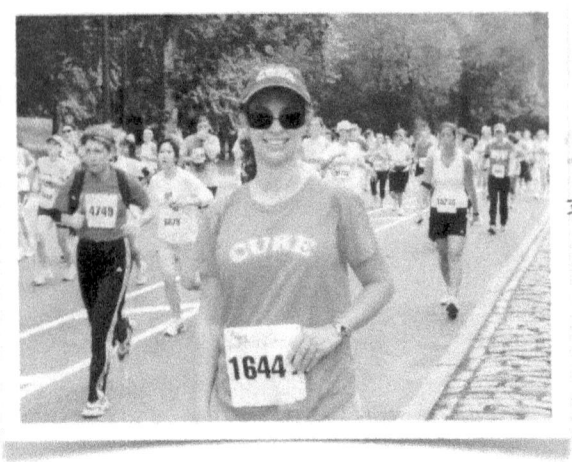
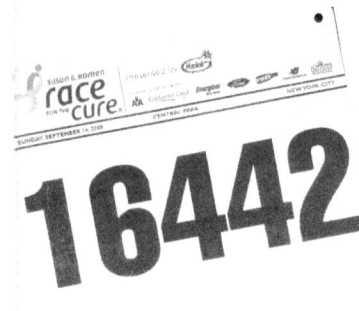

Back on track: participating in the Susan G. Komen Race for the Cure in Central Park in September 2008.

Cancer Society, OncoChat, Network of Strength and the Avon Foundation Breast Cancer Crusade. Thanks to the Internet, women everywhere can connect with each other through these caring support systems.

The Susan G. Komen Foundation sponsors events that not only raise money for breast cancer research, but give survivors opportunities to inspire each other and show the world that the a breast cancer diagnosis is not the end of a woman's story, but just the beginning. I support the Susan G. Komen Race for the Cure in Central Park every year, a five-kilometer walk/run.

Think Positive!

My proactive approach to finding doctors, treatments and the best methods for beating cancer included finding ways to keep a positive attitude and focus on a bright future. Among these was my post-cancer calendar, a list of things I promised to do once I was in recovery. This special calendar, which contained all the things I had to look forward to, became my best friend. While my regular calendar counted down chemotherapy treatments and doctor visits, my post-cancer calendar kept my focus on all the good things to come.

One entry showed the vacation to Jamaica that I would take with my brother and some of our friends. Several weekends were filled with weddings to which I had been invited. I marked the week when I could expect my hair to start growing back and the day that I planned to go back to work. At the end of the year, I filled in that I would have Christmas at my house. My post-cancer calendar helped me have the courage to face the cancer straight on. It became one of the tools for handling the biggest challenge in my life better than I had handled anything else.

Another strategy that helped me keep a positive attitude was helping others. Taking the focus off my chemo and surgeries and putting it on projects that could brighten someone else's life really worked. My friend Leslie helped

While my regular calendar counted down chemotherapy treatments and doctor visits, my post-cancer calendar kept my focus on all the good things to come.

me with one of these activities, giving books to children from families who were less fortunate that our own. We went online to order about 40 copies of Madonna's five children's books, which are fantastic stories for children about friendship and other life lessons. Delivering those beautiful picture books to children and seeing how happy they made them made both of us feel great.

Leslie and I also found a way to help out one of our friends, a young woman who became afflicted with Alopecia, or hair loss, at the age of 25. I knew that my hair would eventually grow back, but we were all aware that hers, unfortunately, would not. Leslie and I pitched in to give her money so that she could have a "procedure" that she really wanted: permanently tattooing her eyebrows.

Having cancer made me believe even more strongly that we should help others, not for the rewards, but because it is the right thing to do. Doing something for a few children and friends and helping several family members in Argentina who were financially in a crunch was easy and reminded me how lucky I am to live in this country. It is easy to forget that we have so much of everything here. God didn't let me die. God protected me and gave me courage. My biggest response was a desire to spread some of that love around in any way I could.

Helping others is a great way to lift your spirits, especially when you're going through a difficult time yourself. I found happiness in babysitting my friends' kids. While in chemotherapy I wasn't going out to dinner often or to clubs. I enjoyed this time with the kids I called my little angels. They were also my biggest fans. Life is such a precious gift, and when you visit a burn unit or a children's cancer ward you will be humbled by their courage and bravery as they try to hold on to life. As I battled cancer I never forgot how much I want children, and that helped me fight. If you feel the same, or you have children, fight! Fight for any dream you have, whether it's meeting the perfect partner or landing a great job. Keep up your spirits, focus on your dreams and fight for them.

Beating cancer is easier if you go out of your way to do something every day that will lift your spirits and find a positive in everything you do. Something as mundane as taking a shower would cheer me up because I learned how to appreciate it. Putting on makeup and treating myself to a cute new jogging outfit did wonders for my attitude.

Painting was another activity that helped me take my mind off my concerns and treatments for a time. For ten years I had driven by a little art store in Brooklyn that had a sign in the window advertising art lessons. One day, after I got cancer, I finally stopped. The owner turned out to be an energetic, fiery man in his 80s who taught the classes himself. Once a week for six months I joined three or four other people and lost myself in the process of painting two photographs that the teacher tore out of a magazine for me. The flowers painting is now hanging in my aunt's house, and the picture of a little lady raking leaves on a farm is in my father's house. I don't claim to be an artist—that wasn't the point—but I did myself a favor by taking an hour or two each week to do something different. It was therapeutic to enter another world where I focused on color and shadows instead of my cancer and listened to that inspiring old man and my fellow students. Studies have shown that any kind of

The Healing Power of Creativity

"Scientific studies tell us that art heals by changing a person's physiology and attitude. The body's physiology changes from one of stress to one of deep relaxation, from one of fear to one of creativity and inspiration.

"Art and music affect every cell in the body instantly to create a healing physiology that changes the immune system and blood flow to all the organs. . . . They create hope and positivity and help people cope with difficulties."

—Michael Samuels, M.D., author of
Spirit Body Healing

creative activity can reduce stress and improve the immune system, so painting was good for my body as well as my mind and spirit.

Sunday has always been my private, personal day, and keeping that routine was another positive approach that helped me get through my ordeal with breast cancer. I loved Sunday as the day to catch up, stay home half the day to read the paper, maybe pamper myself by getting a massage, have brunch with friends and end the day with dinner with my Dad and brother. It didn't matter if it was rainy or sunny, Sundays were my special days. After I got cancer, some Sundays I stayed home and watched movies all day and others I went to church and visited the cemetery, where I talked to my mother and prayed for everyone I love. And some Sundays, I shut out the world and allowed myself to feel sad and have a reflective, solemn day. Making time for all my feelings had a very positive effect.

I discovered that there is great power in staying focused on the positive aspects of life. Every morning when I wake I up and look in the mirror I can say "I choose to be happy today" or "I choose to be worried, afraid and unhappy." It is always a choice. Sometimes we are challenged out of our happy world. But we have the power in our hearts and minds to make choices and come back full circle to happiness. I believe that my soul knows why I am on earth at this point in time and that every

Thoughts To Survive and Thrive By:

- A new ache, pain, medical test or the anniversary of your breast cancer diagnosis may unexpectedly get you down. These feelings are part of being a cancer survivor. But be assured that these emotions will appear further and further apart as you return to your normal life.

- Sadness and grieving for your former healthy self and breasts is not only natural, but an important part of the healing process. Let it out.

- Love yourself and love will come to you.

- Determination is like buying land and envisioning what you would like on your property. I saw myself passing the hurdles of treatment, surgery and staying positive in order to build a beautiful home and my new cancer-survivor life.

- I believe all religions are good. Six years cancer free, I now go to church more than ever to say thank you and pray for everyone I love. Open your heart to love and to whatever religion you choose. You will be ready to face any challenge.

- "Don't sweat the small stuff" are true words to live by. I don't get upset about meetings any more. As a cancer survivor, I have been blessed with a much bigger perspective on life.

challenge that comes my way has a purpose. Which reminds me of a story:

The Teacup

A couple went to England to celebrate their 25th wedding anniversary and shop at a beautiful antique store. They both liked antiques and pottery, especially teacups, and so spotting an exceptional cup, they asked " May we see that? We've never seen a cup so beautiful."

As the lady handed it to them the teacup spoke.

"You don't understand", it said. "I have not always been a teacup. There was a time I was a lump of red clay. My master took me and rolled me, pounded and patted me over and over and I yelled out, 'Don't do that! Leave me alone!" But he only smiled and gently said "Not yet."

"Then, Wham! He placed me on a spinning wheel and I was spun around and around and around. 'Stop it! I'm getting dizzy!' I screamed. But the master only nodded and quietly said 'Not yet.'

"He spun me and poked and prodded and bent me out of shape to suit himself and then - put me in the oven. I had never felt such heat. I yelled and knocked and pounded at the door. 'Help! Get me out of here!'"All he said was. 'Not yet.'

When I thought I couldn't bear it another minute, the door opened. He carefully took me out and placed me on the shelf, where I cooled, waited and wondered what he was going to do to me next. Then suddenly he put me back in the oven. Only it was not like the first time. It was twice as hot and I just knew I would suffocate. I begged, I pleaded, I screamed and I cried. I was convinced I would never make it. Just when I was ready to give up the door opened and he took me out. He put me on the shelf and I began to cool. Oh that felt so good.

"But after I cooled he picked me up and brushed me and painted me all over. The fumes were horrible. 'Oh, please, stop it!' I cried. He only shook his head and said, 'Not yet.'

"An hour later he handed me a mirror and said, 'Look at yourself.' and I did.

"'That's not me!' I said. 'That couldn't be me. It's beautiful. I'm beautiful!'

"Quietly he spoke: 'I want you to remember. It hurt to be rolled and pounded and patted, but had I just left you alone, you would have dried up. I know it made you dizzy to spin around on the wheel, but if I had stopped, you would have crumbled. I know it hurt and it was hot and disagreeable in the oven, but if I hadn't put you in there, you would have cracked. I know the fumes were bad when I brushed and painted you, but if I hadn't done that, you never would have hardened. You would not have any color in your life. And if I hadn't put you back in the oven, you wouldn't have survived for long because the hardness would have not held. Now you are a finished product. Now you are what I had in mind when I first began with you.'"

Every woman feels and reacts differently. Some of my methods may work for you and some may not.

When life seems hard, when you are

136

being pounded and patted and pushed almost beyond endurance; when your world seems to be spinning out of control, when you feel like you are in a fiery furnace of trials, when life seems too hard to bear, try this: brew a cup of your favorite tea in your prettiest teacup, sit down and have a little talk with your potter.

Every woman feels and reacts to things differently. Some of my methods may work for you and some may not. Cut and paste different scenarios to create a custom approach to emotional healing that will work for you. Don't deny yourself a time to be sad; express your feelings and let them flow through you. Pay attention to your need to take things slow. I refused to look at my chest after my first surgery because I wasn't ready yet. Some would call that denial, but I just needed time. I wasn't being weak, just gentle with myself. At that point, ignorance was bliss.

> *"I have found the paradox that if I love until it hurts, then there is no hurt, but only more love."*
>
> —Mother Teresa

❖ Anxiety and sadness are normal and common for women with breast cancer. However, persistent feelings of extreme unhappiness, hopelessness and helplessness, an inability to concentrate and thoughts of death may be symptoms of clinical depression. If you are experiencing those thoughts and feelings, call someone on your medical team. A good overview of the facts on clinical depression can be found at depression-guide.com.

❖ The latest research on therapeutic massage has shown that this treatment is effective in alleviating cancer-related fatigue, easing post-operative pain, boosting the immune system, and decreasing pain and anxiety in hospitalized cancer patients. Nearly one-third of adult Americans report that they have used massage therapy at least once for pain relief. Learn more about therapeutic massage at the website of the American Massage Therapy Association, www.amtamassage.org.

❖ When you go to a massage therapist, tell him/her how many lymph nodes you have had removed, if any, and where they were located. This will help the therapist avoid triggering lymphedema, or swelling. Therapeutic massage is actually very effective in relieving lymphedema, as well.

Chapter 6

BIG GIRLS DO CRY, AND THEN THEY MOVE ON

"Feed your faith and your fears will starve to death."

~Author Unknown

When I received my breast cancer diagnosis and faced the probability of losing my breasts, my second greatest fear, next to dying, was of losing my femininity. Even after I learned how highly advanced reconstruction breast surgery had become since my mother's battle with cancer, I still worried that losing my breasts would make me feel incomplete as a woman. This issue went deep with me because I have always been a very girlie girl.

Throughout my childhood I loved playing with dolls, decorating my dollhouses and reading fashion magazines to develop my taste in clothes. I never outgrew my love of playing dress up, and when I was in my teens I had a terrific opportunity to indulge that passion. One of my mother's close friends worked in a high-end women's boutique on Madison Avenue called Soleil. She let me visit the shop whenever I liked, and I spent many afternoons trying on sparkly, sequined dresses that cost thousands of dollars apiece. That helped make up for the role model I had at home in my stepmother, my father's second wife. She was on the frumpy side, and her chain smoking and love of whisky highballs didn't help. But thanks to my mother's friend and others, I grew to love feminine things. Diana, one of my cousins from Argentina who is about ten years older that I am, was a big help in this way. She always treated me like an adult by talking to me like an equal and asking for my opinion on things, which made me feel great about myself. Because I didn't grow up with a

> *"Maintaining a positive body-image is an important part of the healing process. What you wear on the outside can impact how you feel on the inside. Clothes are not only functional; they can also change your mood, lift your spirits, and provide you with a creative outlet. And since getting dressed is part of a daily routine anyway, why not use your clothing as a tool to feel good about yourself?"*
>
> —Emily Spivak, founder of Shop Well with You: A Body-Image Resource for Women Surviving Cancer

Mom, she was the first person I ever saw with a French manicure. She was a classy young woman and I wanted to mimic all her feminine qualities. When I was fifteen she came to visit and we all went out to dinner. She brought me a gift, a bottle of Ralph Lauren perfume, which

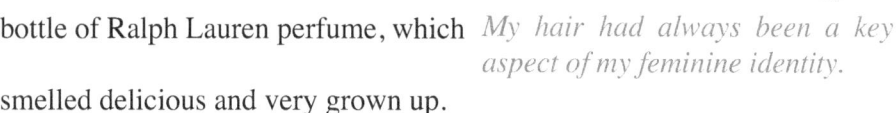

My hair had always been a key aspect of my feminine identity.

smelled delicious and very grown up.

It made me feel so special, and it is still one of my favorite scents.

Retaining Your Feminine Identity

For me, femininity went hand in hand with dignity. When I went through chemotherapy, I wanted to keep looking beautiful on the outside and feeling beautiful on the inside. I hoped that people would not pass judgment on me when I lost my hair. I considered myself a person who would not judge people who looked "different" just because their appearance strayed from the norm. But I hadn't considered how hard it would be to keep from doing that very thing to myself. When I first looked at my powder-white, bald head, I told myself that cancer was just part of me and did not define me. I knew that I should continue to be confident about my looks and not worry about what other people thought. Those were noble ideas to live by, but it took some time to actually get there.

Getting dressed and putting on makeup every day while going through cancer treatment may not be easy at first. It took me awhile to put my own advice into practice after I started chemo. As girly as I was, I lost my motivation to look good for awhile and wore pajamas and slippers everywhere. I just didn't care. I had four closets full of beautiful clothes, but I was a bit depressed and my body image was the last thing on my mind. My girlfriend Ivette tried to snap me out of it by setting me up with one of her friends. He called me several times and I kept canceling, but he was persistent and after about the tenth call I agreed to meet him for coffee. I didn't expect him to be anything special, partly because I wasn't in the mood and partly because I thought Ivette had set up the blind date with any old guy just to get me out of the house. Anxious to get it over with, I threw on a pair of green plaid flannel pajamas and black, furry Payard boots. I didn't bother to put on makeup or do anything with my fuzzy mess of hair. What a mistake! James turned out to be extremely handsome and funny. We had a good conversation, but I don't think he felt sparks. I couldn't blame him, because my personality was about as dazzling as my outfit. It was too bad, because Jim had potential.

When I told Ivette how awful I looked and what a lousy first impression I must have made, she died laughing because it was so unlike me. If Jim saw me on the street today he wouldn't recognize me because I never look like that. But I wasn't ready to pull myself together at that point. Jim told Ivette that he wasn't going to call me again because he could tell that I wasn't interested. I forgave myself and let it go.

The moral of my blind date story is that it is worthwhile to make the effort to pick yourself up and get out in the world, even when you don't feel great. You never know who may be ready to cross your path and add some positive energy to your life.

It would take a little time to talk myself into dressing nicely and wearing makeup when I left the house, but once I did it made a big difference in my attitude. Looking good gave me a shot of confidence and made me feel more comfortable about interacting with people.

Before I got cancer, my vibrant, energetic, humorous and outgoing personality guaranteed that I would get attention wherever I went. My life wasn't perfect, but I was happy, and when you are happy you attract people. High energy and

"Be who you are and say what you feel because those who mind don't matter, and those who matter don't mind"
Dr. Seuss

Caring for Your Feminine Side

To nurture a strong connection to your womanly self while undergoing breast cancer treatment, try to:

* Pamper yourself with visits to a spa, free makeup consultations at a department store, pedicures and manicures and new clothes

* Wear makeup and dress nicely—don't stay in your pajamas or sweats for days on end!

* Enjoy having the time to catch up on good books and movies

* Keep a journal to write about your thoughts, feelings, experiences, the people in your life and plans for the future

* Start a hobby like photography, drawing or painting, sewing or crocheting, pottery, learning a musical instrument or writing poetry. I took up cooking, which included taking classes and getting hooked on the Food Network. It was good for me and *great* for my friends and family!

* Take a class in something that has always interested you, such as a wine course, local history, art or music appreciation, a language, world religions or making pastry. Many towns offer a wide variety of classes through community organizations like the YMCA, and the college nearest you may offer extension courses.

* Sign up for yoga, ballet, Pilates or other classes at your local health club or YMCA.

* Listen to good music

* Join a book group, or start one with your friends. Many publishers provide book group discussion guides on their websites.

* Hang out with friends to watch movies or just talk. Surround yourself with positive people.

laughter are contagious, and I loved to flirt, in a good way. But when I began feeling worn out from chemo and got in the habit of leaving the house in pajamas, the attention stopped. I may have been blessed with good looks, but they were hard to find beneath my ghost-pale complexion, messy short hair and baggy clothes. Instead of drawing smiles and chit-chat when I walked down the street or through a store, people turned away or ignored me completely. Construction workers stopped yelling out sweet nothings.

I missed the attention and the positive energy that I had always found in places like my favorite home warehouse store, where I loved to get decorating ideas and dream about the house I would have one day. Previously I would find myself surrounded by friendly salespeople who were eager to help, but when I walked through the aisles looking tired and grungy, I was virtually invisible. I could have tried to carry a bathtub out of there by myself and no one would have noticed me. In spite of that, I got a lift out of shopping there while I was undergoing chemotherapy.

Like my mother, who bought all kinds of crazy things

"Body-image is not how people see you, but how you perceive yourself. Wear clothes that make you feel comfortable and confident."

—Emily Spivak

from the infomercials she watched on TV, I felt good buying things for my future house. While I was undergoing chemo, I bought an electric fireplace, patio furniture and a stainless steel gas barbecue grill, all of which had to put in a rented storage unit because I had no room for them in my two-bedroom apartment. Buying these items for my dream home helped me see the glass half full and gave me a positive attitude about the future. And not every visit was an alienating experience. One day, when I showed up at the store in a wig and big Chanel sunglasses, a clerk was convinced that I was Julia Roberts or some other actress trying to go about her business incognito. As he wheeled my cart out to my car, I felt happy that he had no idea that I was bald and had tissue expanders in my chest. He begged me to tell him who I was and promised not to tell anyone, which really made my day.

My girlfriend Nazy, who lives in California, also helped draw me out of my slump during chemotherapy by visiting me several times and working hard to cheer me up. One night, as we were leaving my place to go out to dinner, she refused to let me walk out the door in my pajamas. She was all decked out and insisted that it was my turn to do the same. I trudged back to my room and put on a nice pair of jeans and a top and some makeup. Feeling nice clothes on my body and seeing some color in

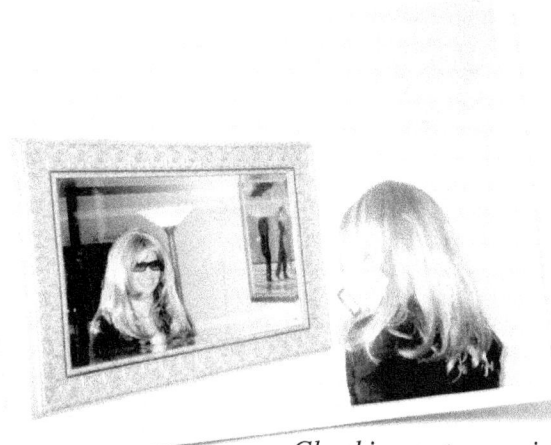

*Checking out my quirky blonde wig, which I
wore a few times just for fun.*

my face did wonders. I turned a corner that night and never wore my

pajamas out of the house again.

When you feel good about yourself you attract people. Energy is

everything. I began to feel better about myself and it showed. I started

going out on dates again, even though I was still undergoing

chemotherapy. I wasn't interested in getting into a serious relationship yet,

but having someone flirt with me was fun.

When I felt drained from chemo, just taking a shower every day

was enough to lift my spirits. But it was my habit of walking regularly that

made the biggest difference in my strength and healthiness. Throughout

my adult life my doctors had stressed the importance of exercise for cardio

health, and after my cancer diagnosis my oncologist Dr. Chuang emphasized that exercise was especially important during chemotherapy. Because the medications can make cancer patients dizzy and nauseous, walking is vital for improving circulation, pumping oxygen through the body and increasing overall energy.

Others, like my brother, walked with me for as long as I wanted. My friend Claudia always pushed me to go a little further, which helped me learn how strong I really was. I sensed that I was working the toxins out of my body as I walked and looked at the flowers, watched the old men play bocce ball, passed strolling couples and made room for rollerblades to whiz by. I was part of the living. The people around me probably didn't make a big deal out of their visits to the park, but for me every walk was a big accomplishment. All of my friends got used to the fact that visiting me meant going to the park, and three of them in particular couldn't even keep up with me. I was walking for my life.

Losing—and Regaining Your

Crowning Glory

My hair has also played a big role in my feminine identity. My second

> *The people around me probably didn't make a big deal out of their visits to the park, but for me every walk was a big accomplishment. I was walking for my life.*

chemotherapy treatment hurt the most—mentally and emotionally—because I knew that a week or two later my hair would start falling out. Until then I had been able to stand in front of the mirror in my underwear and mastectomy bra and feel whole, like myself. But when it came to being brave about fighting cancer, my hair was my Achilles heel. I would have done anything not to lose it. I loved my long hair, and the thought of being bald reminded me of my mother's transformation from a beauty to a bald, frail and very sick woman. Like a scarlet letter, my bald head would soon mark me as an outcast. Strangers in the street would be able to tell what was going on with me. I grieved for this future loss, but I knew I had good reason to be sad and I did not take anti-depressants.

Allowing my grief to flow naturally ultimately gave me the strength to be grateful and filled with hope as I counted down the last weeks of my chemotherapy. I was ready to live with the fact that four cycles of chemo would result in temporary hair loss. The medication destroys some healthy cells, specifically the fastest-growing cells, like hair follicles. The chemo medication targets these structures because, like cancer cells, they divide quickly: once every one to three days.

One of my closest friends told me that wrapping ice packs around my head would prevent this side effect. "I wish," I told myself, because I knew that this was a myth. My friend, who is a doctor himself, was just trying to help because he knew how terrible I felt about losing my hair. Dr Chuang had filled me in on all the facts about chemotherapy, including the common myths about how to avoid certain side effects. Unfortunately, nothing has yet been developed that can combat the hair loss. But I stuck to the facts and knew that going bald for a few months was a small price to pay. After giving my feelings their due, I felt stronger and realized that being alive would be an amazing and fair tradeoff for the temporary loss of my hair.

Once I made peace with that fact, I decided to make the best of it. In mid-June, 2005, just before starting my second chemotherapy treatment, I had my hair shaved and donated the long, brown tresses to Locks of Love, the non-profit organization that provides hairpieces for financially disadvantaged children with long-term medical hair loss.

My stylist at Paul Anthony Aesthetics in Manhasset, New York, took his time and listened as I tearfully shared my feelings about my upcoming hair loss. The entire staff was thoughtful and compassionate, which made it an unforgettable experience. Several of my guy friends showed me their love and support by shaving their heads at the same time. My girlfriends Ivette and Nazy offered to shave their beautiful hair off,

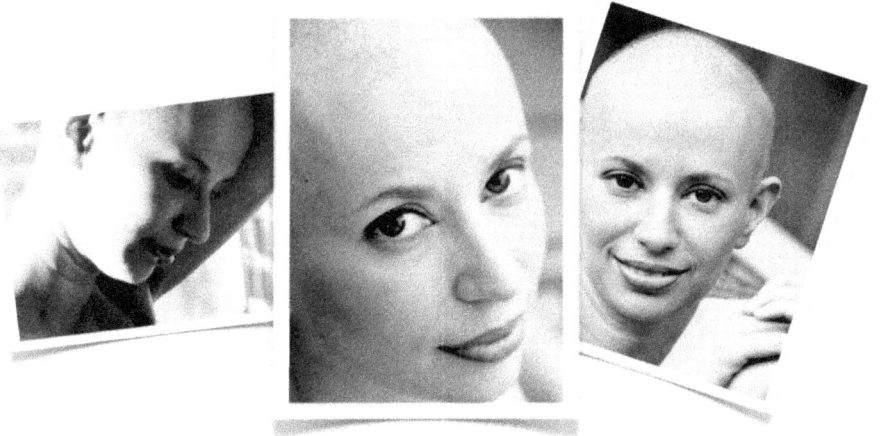

Before my second chemotherapy treatment, I had my head shaved.

too, and Ivette planned to make a wig for me with hers. I appreciated their willingness to make this sacrifice for my sake, but I talked them out of it.

I strongly recommend that you be proactive and shave your hair before it begins to fall out. If you choose to do this and donate your healthy hair to Locks of Love, you will not only save yourself the trauma of seeing your hair come out in chunks, but you will also feel the joy of helping a child endure a serious illness with dignity. It is a brave and beautiful thing to do.

It was exciting to discover that wigs are much more natural looking than they were in my mother's day. My insurance only covered the purchase of one at less than $200, but I bought five of them in various styles and colors. At one shop, I was taken into a private room where my stylist brought me a selection to try on. Among them was a beautiful

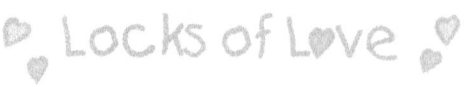

Being proactive by cutting your hair before it falls out will save you emotional trauma. In addition, if you donate your hair to Locks of Love, you will feel the joy of knowing you helped a child endure a serious illness with dignity.

creation made from real, unprocessed hair, ready to wear for a whopping

price of $3,600. I called my voice of reason, Anne, and described the wig

to her. She thought I was nuts to entertain spending that amount of money

and suggested I wear it for a while to see if it would restore my

confidence. I followed her advice and sat in the private room for a few

minutes, looking at myself in the mirror and playing with the soft strands

of hair. It didn't make me feel any more confident than the less expensive

models, and the experiment helped me learn that confidence has to come

from within. I decided I would rather use the money for the Jamaica trip

that I had scheduled on my post-cancer calendar.

Scarves are another option until your hair begins to grow out. I wore them frequently because my wigs felt too hot on many summer days. Chemo in the summer was a tough combination, but now and then an unexpected act of kindness made it easier.

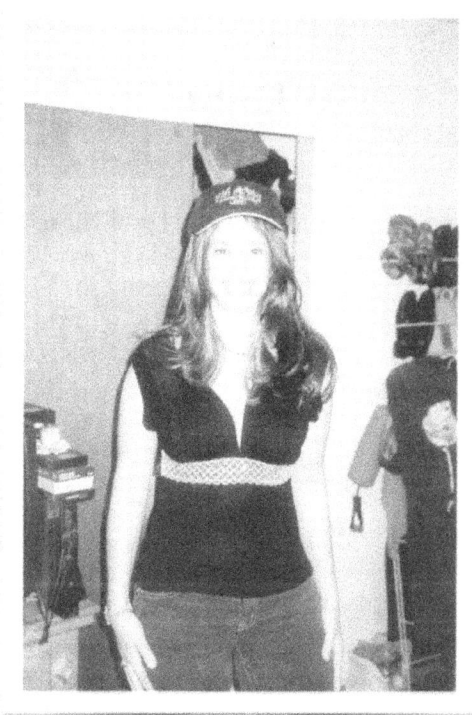

Wearing one of my favorite wigs under a baseball cap. It almost looked like my own hair.

One hot evening, I got ready to go out to dinner at one of my favorite restaurants, the posh River Café in Brooklyn, with my brother and two uncles who were visiting from Argentina. I put on a black dress that looked beautiful on my slender chemo figure. I planned on wearing one of my favorite wigs, one that resembled my hair before I lost it. Uncle Claudio thought it was ridiculous for me to suffer on such a hot night with a wig. He refused to go out to dinner with us if I wore it, so I finally agreed to leave it home and go with a bare head.

Wigging Out: Tips on Hair Coverings

- When you visit a wig shop, bring along some pictures of you in a hairstyle you love so the stylist can visualize what you want. Or choose photos from a magazine, describe a celebrity hairstyle you like or ask what kind of style he/she recommends for your features.

- A wig cap, which costs about three dollars, helps makes the wig feel more comfortable and gives a more natural-looking fit.

- The hair stylist I worked with in New York suggested placing a gel band around my head, beneath the wig, to keep my head cool. It helped tremendously.

- If it's not convenient for you to drop off your wig for a wash and style, ask the salon if you can mail it overnight and have it returned the same way. You could also ask a friend to drop it off and pick it up for you.

- It is helpful to have a backup wig to wear while the other is being cleaned and restyled.

- Hairpieces designed to be worn beneath a scarf, cap or hat are great alternatives to a full wig.

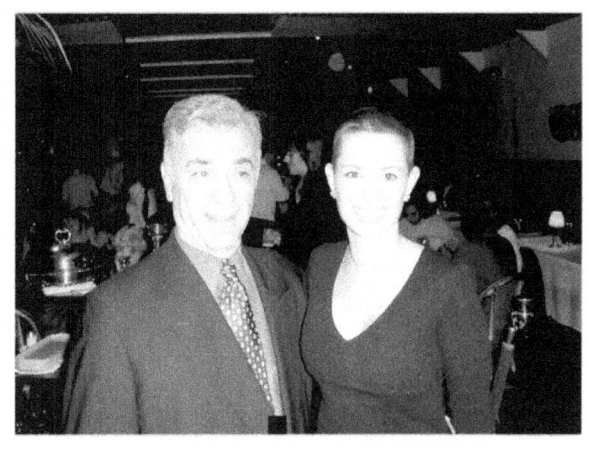

Nearly bald and out on the town with
Uncle Claudio at the River Cafe.

As I walked into the elegant dining room that overlooked the East River and the Manhattan skyline, I was sure that everyone was staring at me. I was horrified to imagine what they were thinking and wanted to run out and never come back. Then Victor, our waiter, came to the table and commented on how beautiful I looked. He had sensed my discomfort and went out of his way to put me at ease. His polite yet very warm and caring words made me relax and I had a wonderful evening. The experience was so freeing that I rarely wore wigs after that and instead had fun with my look. And every time I see Victor at the River Café I say hello and thank him for helping me through that difficult situation.

When I did wear a wig, I felt a bit more normal. On the Fourth of July, another hot night, I wore a wig to a party that I attended with three good friends. No one else at the party knew that I had cancer and I didn't want to shake them up. The wig must have looked pretty good because a few guys talked to me quite a bit and some even flirted with me. It was a pleasant surprise because even though I looked all right, I felt weak and out of it and my self-confidence was still pretty low. I was also nervous because people were jumping in the swimming pool and I was afraid that someone would throw me in and my wig would fall off. My friends took care of that by staying close and protecting me. Afterward, in the car on the way home, I finally took off my wig. We parked the car on my block and I started walking to my apartment. When I got in front of the building, I plopped it back on my head, backwards, and stood there grinning like a troll. I freaked out a few neighbors who walked by, but my friends were so tired that they didn't even notice until they got close enough to say good night.

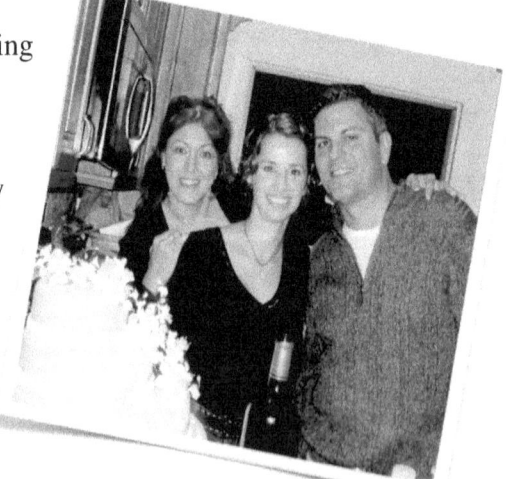

Celebrating life with my friends Daisy and Rob, I'm sporting a short, wavy hairdo about six months after my last chemo treatment. The cake was a tribute to my Mom's love of lavish cakes.

I finished chemotherapy on July 29th. By the time I returned to work in October I had packed away my wigs for good and was feeling great in my super-short do.

Losing my hair was the toughest part of my journey with breast cancer, more traumatizing than having a double mastectomy and going through months of chemotherapy. As shallow as it may sound, I felt that my beautiful locks defined me as a woman. But my sense of loss didn't last long. I received many compliments on my short hairstyle and people who didn't know me never guessed the battle I had just won. This inspired me to encourage my mentor and friend, Greta, to stop wearing her wigs, too, and she agreed. She received the same positive feedback on her short hair and was much more comfortable.

I returned to work on October 6th, ready to hit the ground running at an important plan-of-action meeting. I was ecstatic to be back, and everyone at the company made it one of the best days of my life by acknowledging my courage and welcoming me back with a standing ovation.

I can truly say that the breast cancer experience was worth it. Not only for saving my life, but for giving me a new appreciation

Your hair begins to grow back about two to three weeks after your final chemo treatment.

Post-Cancer Hair Care

- Most physicians advise you to avoid coloring your hair for six months after your treatments end. You may try a temporary (vegetable-based) rinse to brighten or enhance your color, which usually lasts for a few weeks.

- During your treatment, looking as healthy as possible will help lift your spirits. Moisturize your entire body, including your scalp. I splurged on high-end products, especially for my face, such as Shisheido-Bio Performance. If that's not an option for you, more economical brands like Nivea also work well.

- If you temporarily lose your eyebrows, I recommend a Chanel pencil to fill them in. It works like magic—you cannot tell that your brows are penciled in. Go to the Chanel counter at a department store and ask the salesperson to suggest a pencil color for your brows to compliment your coloring. I still use my pencil to enhance my eyebrows, which grew back in after chemo just like my hair.

- Your skin tone will probably change due to medications and chemotherapy, so you will need new makeup. Drop by the cosmetic counter at your favorite store and get a makeup consultation to find out which colors and products work best for you. Before chemo I loved bronzes on my cheeks, but my skin became much lighter from the treatments and I made the change to pinks.

- Take good care of your hair with gentle shampoos and regular conditioning. Healthy hair should grow about six inches a year.

- Ask someone with a great haircut for a referral.

- Treat yourself to blowouts (professional blow-drying done in sections with conditioners) at the salon for a few months to keep your hair looking great while it grows out.

- A good stylist can help you experiment and have fun with your growing hair. I learned how to use gel and cute barrettes to come up with adorable styles.

- If you can't wait to have long hair again, you can invest in extensions. They are made from real hair and can be woven in without any artificial materials. Extensions are expensive, but they're gorgeous and last for several months before needing to be re-attached closer your scalp as your hair grows.

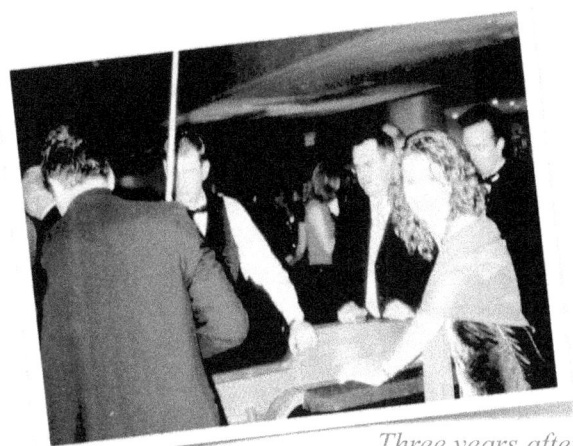

Three years after breast cancer, I'm back in the game and life

for every precious day and learning about the power of a positive attitude and being surrounded by loving support. I had a double mastectomy and lost my hair for a few months, but after all was said and done I survived it and now feel more like a woman than ever. I'm back at the beach in my bikini and I feel sexy naked. It's a beautiful thing! After all the fear and pain, I earned my vanity. I deserve to be proud of my body and of everything else that makes me Judy, a woman.

Tips

❖ To learn more about the research on the beneficial effects of
acupuncture during breast cancer treatment, read "Acupuncture Eases
Breast Cancer Treatment Side Effects," *Washington Post,* September
22, 2008, found at www.washingtonpost.com/ wp-dyn/content/article/
2008/09/22/AR2008092200793.html.

❖ Check out the guidelines for donating hair to Locks of Love on the
organization's website, locksoflove.org.

❖ Learn variations for wearing head scarves, turbans and hats from Look
Good . . . Feel Better, a wonderful website for women dealing with
cancer found at www.lookgoodfeelbetter.org.

My dear friend, Ram Aeri, created a message of hope by writing this lovely prose poem for me:

The Butterfly
by Ram Aeri

Once upon a time there was a bed of beautiful flowers in the middle of a meadow. They were pink, blue, crimson, yellow, orange, all kinds that you can think of. They all looked very majestic, swinging back and forth in a playful manner with every burst of the spring breeze. One day, a gust of wind brought a surprise visitor, a beautiful butterfly from a faraway land. The flowers had never seen anything like this before. The visitor was delighted to have companions who were equally as beautiful as she, and seemed too gleeful in their midst, as if they were waiting for her. Like them she was full of life, always hopping from here to there in an obliging display of her gliding charm. Sunshine and cool breezes helped choreograph this dazzling show and it went on ceaselessly, unmindful of the passing of the time.

One day, a storm of thick dark clouds formed overhead and the next Moment a heavy downpour pelted everything under it with a merciless fury. The delicate butterfly could not fight the mighty rain and fell to the ground. She tried to get up again and again, but to no avail. The wings felt too heavy to move. Once a queen in the air, there she was, lying flattened and lifeless on her wings in the muddy water. She thought it was all over; her companions were sad and helpless. It seemed dark and she felt hopeless.

All of a sudden, the rain stopped and the sky started to clear. All the water was gone and the sun broke out through the clouds, warming up things below. Soon her wings began to dry and she started to feel her strength. The breeze helped by getting under her wings and giving her an initial lift. Soon the gliding beauty, with a burst of fresh vigor, was flying again. A beautiful rainbow above in the sky joined in this colorful show of nature underneath. There was a smile on everybody's face. Happy days were here again. Nobody could have imagined life any better than this.

Chapter 7

THE NAKED TRUTH

"Sex with its joy clears and sharpens the vision."
—Helen Keller

I have always considered sex an important part of good health. A healthy sex life has many advantages. With my lifestyle—from the hustle and bustle of getting to work in the city to dealing with a high-energy job all day and then running home to handle my other responsibilities and commitments—sex gives me some balance. Sex with your partner can make you forget about the bad part of your day or celebrate the good.

Michael and I had a great sex life, before and after my breast cancer diagnosis. There is nothing like loving and being touched by your partner. When I got sick, all the rubbish about diets and worrying about my figure went out the window. Michael loved me, all of me, as I was.

With all the changes my body went through, from surgeries to chemotherapy, he continued to be all over me. He never stopped looking at me like I was hot and amazing, and we had sex throughout my treatments. There were days when we just held each other because I felt horrible from chemo, but the physical contact was wonderful. Sex helped me restore my sense of femininity and filled me with a strong, loving feeling that made me feel like I could face anything.

Sex and Healing

In my darkest hours I saw myself as bald and weak, but Michael

Physical affection has an enormously positive effect on the body. It's a medical fact that kissing and hugging can help cure just about anything!

never lost sight of the finished product. Through it all, I was the same girl he had always been crazy about. Cancer didn't beat me and it didn't take away one ounce of my sexuality.

Some women consider sex a chore or a reward for their other half. I consider it a reward for me. Sexually, I still felt good about my self when I had breast cancer. Wearing a top to bed for a few months, until I had healed from my reconstructive surgery, made me feel as sexy as I did before I got cancer.

No matter how lousy I felt due to chemotherapy or other medications, I continued to enjoy sex and knew that it was helping me on many levels. Physical affection has an enormously positive effect on the body. It's a medical fact that kissing and hugging can help cure just about anything!

Even though Michael and I broke up before I finished chemotherapy, we remained friends and continued to sleep together from time to time. I was bald, fatigued and not in the mood to look for a relationship, so I continued to be intimate with Michael for several months. Again, sex is a great distraction and helped me connect more to the normalcy of life. It may not sound rational that we broke up yet still loved each other and remained intimate, but that's what worked for us. We stopped arguing and just had fun. I felt like a ton of bricks had been lifted off my shoulders.

I was fortunate to have a partner who was very comfortable having sex throughout my treatment, but in reality breast cancer can take a toll on many women's sex lives. Many of the breast cancer survivors I talked to preferred not to be active with their partners during chemotherapy. All of them said that they were very tired, and for some of them this was enough to turn them off to sex. Fatigue can easily affect a woman's sex drive even

The Top 10 Health Benefits of Sex

Medical studies have proven that sex is good for you. Based on scientific evidence, we know for a fact that:

1. **Sex Relieves Stress:** Researchers have found that sex reduces blood pressure and other stress-related factors. In women, there is a *proven link* between hugs and lower blood pressure!

2. **Sex Enhances Immunity:** "Frequent" sex—once or twice a week—keeps the doctor away by increasing levels of immunoglobulin A, or IgA, an antibody that can protect from getting colds and infections. Healthy moderation is the key. One study showed that those who have sex once or twice a week produce more IgA than those who are abstinent, have sex less frequently OR have sex *more* often than twice a week.

3. **Sex Burns Calories:** One-half hour of sex burns at least 85 calories. Enough said.

4. **Sex Is Good for the Heart:** Studies show that having sex twice a week is good for cardiovascular health.

5. **Sex Improves Self-Esteem:** Making love is a proven way to boost how good you feel about yourself.

6. **Sex Deepens Intimacy:** Sexual activity boosts our drive to nurture and bond by increasing levels of oxytocin, the "love hormone," which enhances our ability to form bonds and build trust with others.

7. **Sex Reduces Pain:** The rise in oxytocin that comes from having sex triggers an increase in endorphins, nature's pain relievers. One study showed that increased oxytocin levels lowered participants' pain thresholds by more than half. Doesn't that sound like more fun than taking an aspirin?

8. **Sex Lowers the Risk of Prostate Cancer:** An extra benefit for men to keep in mind.

9. **Sex Strengthens Pelvic Muscles:** Tightening pelvic floor muscles, also called a basic Kegel exercise, increases pleasure during sex and lowers the risk of incontinence later in life.

10. **Sex Improves Sleep:** Raising oxytocin levels by having sex has yet another benefit: promoting sleep. Deep, restful sleep is essential for psychological health, maintaining the immune system, allowing the body to repair tissue and much more.

Source: WebMD.com

when she's healthy, so feeling uninterested in sex due to fatigue from chemo is a common issue. Chemo just knocks you out.

I met Dr Ruth, the nationally known sex expert, at an Erectile Dysfunction Symposium that I attended for work. I was about thirty years old at the time and asked her to share some pearls of wisdom with me. Through the years I've never forgotten her advice:

- Explore!
- You are in control—sex is what you make it!
- Sex is not a four-letter word.
- The #1 sex organ is your brain.

In terms of women going through breast cancer, I think that Dr. Ruth's most important point is that the brain is our biggest erogenous zone. Breast cancer brings up body image and femininity issues that can turn us away from our sexuality, so it's important to remember that there is much more to our sexuality than specific body parts. Don't let cancer take anything more than it does.

Sexuality is a Decision-Making Factor for Women with Breast Cancer

The aesthetic details of the breast is not a priority for some survivors that I spoke to, and that's understandable. On the other hand, some women I met considered breast sensation so important that they decided to do whatever it took to preserve their breasts. In most cases, that meant neoadjuvant (initial) chemo before surgery to shrink the tumor so that only part of the breast was removed in a lumpectomy or partial mastectomy. Neither was a choice for me because I wanted to be more certain about best outcomes. The breast cancer survivors I spoke to who were over age 40 and carried the mutated BRAC gene chose to have their ovaries and their breasts removed in order to guarantee, as much as possible, cancer recurrence.

Sexual Side Effects of Chemotherapy

Physical. Some chemotherapy drugs can cause a temporary or permanent loss of estrogen, which can lead to vaginal thinning or dryness. These conditions can make intercourse painful. When the ovaries stop functioning, you also lose testosterone, the "hormone of desire," which may also lower your sex drive. Lubricants, vaginal estrogen and acupuncture can help treat these side effects.

Psychological. The fatigue, hair loss, nausea, weight loss or gain that accompanies chemotherapy may make you feel unattractive and lower your desire for sex. Every activity you do to brighten your mood and make your days easier will also make you feel more comfortable being close to your partner.

Sexual Issues with Chemo

A breast cancer diagnosis can make you think that you are too sick, depressed or just too preoccupied with the illness to have sex. Side effects of chemotherapy and of the disease itself can also affect your attitude toward and experience of sex. This does not mean that you must sacrifice your sexuality to cancer. At the first sign of lower sex drive, painful intercourse or other sexual issues during your treatment, talk to members of your medical team. Don't be shy about bringing up these issues, because there are treatments to offset some of them, such as vaginal estrogen for the dryness that may result from chemotherapy. Other breast cancer survivors can also provide advice on the sexual side effects of treatment. If you are not comfortable talking about this with other women in a support group setting, go online to a chat or forum where you can remain anonymous. A good place to start is the American Cancer Society's Cancer Survivors Network. In addition to seeking help from your doctors and support network, talk to your partner about your sexual concerns.

I had never considered breast cancer stimulation very important for enjoying sex, but I'm glad that I finally made the choice to have this final, cosmetic procedure because my breasts look so incredibly natural.

Plan ahead for this important conversation and arrange a sleepover for the children and/or cuddle up somewhere comfortable. Take it slow, and make time for intimacy.

Love and Connect with Your Healing Body

Once I felt ready to start dating again I wanted to reconnect even more with my feminine side. After a little research on exercise programs that would help me feel sexy in my healthy new body, I discovered a new type of workout designed exactly for that. The S Factor is a striptease-like workout for women that focuses on sensual movements.

Complete with pole-dancing moves, which S Factor founder and actress Sheila Kelley calls "ballet on a pole," this workout was exactly what I needed. Each women-only class was held in low lighting with no mirrors so that we felt uninhibited to swirl our hips and move with sensuality. The moves were a gentle combination of ballet, yoga and Pilates, and I always got a full, strenuous workout. I looked forward to those two-hour sessions like crazy, and they really paid off by giving me more self-confidence, inner peace, erotic power and a great body.

Dance and movement classes are springing up all over the country to address the physical and emotional needs of breast cancer survivors.

Women are also reconnecting with their femininity and sexuality by taking belly dancing lessons at a studio or with a DVD at home. Two dance programs, created by breast cancer survivors, that are expanding to hospitals and cities around the country are The Lebed Method and Moving On Aerobics.

The Lebed Method: Focus on Healing Through Movement and Dance was designed to help breast cancer survivors increase their range of movement and boost their sense of femininity and sexuality. I love the

Keep It Intimate

➤ **Communicate!** Tell your partner how you feel about your sex life and what you would like to change. You might want to talk about your concerns, your beliefs about why your sex life is the way it is, your feelings, and what would make you feel better.

➤ **Approaching it openly** avoids blame, stays positive, and gives your partner a better sense of how you are feeling.

➤ **Be proud of your body.** It got you through treatment!

➤ **Think of things that help you feel more attractive and confident.**

➤ **Focus on the positive.** Try to be aware of your thoughts, since they can affect your sex life.

➤ **Touch each other.** Kiss, hug, and cuddle, even if you cannot have the kind of sex that you used to have.

➤ **Be open to change.** You may find new ways to enjoy intimacy

Source: National Cancer Institute, www.cancer.gov

program's motto: "Surviving is Important . . . But Thriving Is Elegant!"

Moving On Aerobics: Joyful Dance Exercise for Breast Cancer Survivors was created by a breast cancer survivor who wanted to share the healing effects of dance with other women. Allison Stern Rosen, Ph.D., a psychologist and co-founder of the program, described how movement helped her find her way back to joyful living while she was recovering from breast cancer surgery and treatment:

> *Sitting around, depressed and lethargic, my one solace was music. It cheered me up. One day, I began dancing to the music. Although, it hurt to walk, I could sway and rock. At last, I had discovered a way to regain my strength. Joy is too calm a word to describe what I felt. I had a future again.*

Acupuncture Can Ease Chemo

Acupuncture, the ancient Chinese treatment that uses very slender needles to unblock the body's energy flow, can ease the side effects of chemotherapy that result from a loss of estrogen.

In one medical study, acupuncture was just as effective as antidepressant drugs in relieving the menopausal-like symptoms of women being treated for breast cancer, but it had no side effects and was longer lasting.

The Dating Challenge During and After Recovery

A few months after my last chemotherapy treatment Michael and I took our long-awaited trip to Jamaica with some friends. By that time we wanted to give ourselves one last opportunity to see if we could reconnect as a couple and move into a serious relationship. We loved each other a lot, but were also able to hurt each other so much. The vacation was wonderful, but we realized that there was no turning back for us. We knew that we deserved more than just settling for the familiar, so we made real closure with each other. There was no doubt that we would still be friends —close friends—but it was time to move on and keep things very simple with each other. When I got home, I was ready to start looking for someone to share my life with. Michael and I remained friends but we didn't sleep together any more. I was happy, healthy and the owner a new house that I bought to launch the start of my new, cancer-free life.

Facing the dating scene after breast cancer posed new challenges for me. I knew that I would be upfront about my cancer story, but I had no idea how a man would handle the information. As I gathered courage to get back out in the world and meet strangers, I recalled the Dalai Lama's words: 'Take into account that great love and great achievements involve great risk."

Some of my friends thought that I shared too much when I started dating. Did I really need to tell guys right away that I had cancer? Physically, the cancer was gone (although I would be monitored for years), but some of the emotional effects were—and are—still there. They

Move Your Body: Dance Can Heal!

A study written up in *Cancer Nursing* in 2005 discussed the improved quality of life in a group of breast cancer survivors who participated in therapeutic dance classes. The article explains that dance has been part of the healing process since the earliest times:

"The roots of dance in healing go back to ancient societies in which dance rituals frequently accompanied major life changes. Dancing, religion, music, and medicine were inseparable in the early years of civilization. [One researcher] proposed that dance may help the healing process as a person gains a sense of control through

(a) spiritual components of dance;

(b) mastery of movement;

(c) escape from stress and pain by a change in emotion, states of consciousness, and/or physical capability; and

(d) confronting stressors."

do not feel like baggage, however. The cancer period in my life is a part of me, and I am not ashamed of what I have been through. The answer I had for my friends was, if a man can't see past that and see all the attributes I bring to the table, then he is definitely not worth getting to know!

I went out on a lot of dates, just chatting and getting to know new people. There was no kissing or intimacy because I never felt any sparks. I am a tough cookie. There were opportunities, but for me, sex is meant to be with someone special. I was ready for a new chapter to begin and I knew that I had to wait for everything to feel just right. I didn't have to wait long.

Life is full of surprises. I had first met Brandon about three years ago. My dear friend Jessica met Brandon on a plane ride back from vacation. She had a hunch that we would click. She invited him to a dinner party at my house. She thought it would be an informal and fun way to meet. I don't know who was more shy, Brandon or me. Jessica was right on the money. We clicked instantly. He sent me a box of chocolate duds with a note in the mail the following day. The duds was a reference not to judge him initially. He was getting divorced so he was missing his swagger. Brandon didn't know he never lost it. I found him handsome, genuine and so funny. "You know you're in love when you can't fall asleep because reality is better than your dreams." Dr Seuss.

My heart told me it was happy. I know I'm a better person because of him. Living life with my heart wide open.

Over the years, my friends have teased me about being very confident professionally, but never a risk taker in the romantic department. My friends are happy to see me with a pulse, back in the game. I love the feeling of being in love. It feels like the first day of fall. I am opening my heart again and trying. I don't know what our future holds, but I am enjoying my "right now" and appreciate all I have.

As I write this I am six years cancer free and I feel confident and beautiful. I am still finding balance and harmony inside myself, but I have my life back. If you are single, dare to put yourself out there again and look for a partner. If you are married, hang on and love one another because when you beat cancer together there will be nothing tougher to encounter in the future. I recently listened to my friend Elaine, who is also three years cancer free, argue with her husband over the color of granite they should choose for their kitchen. They couldn't agree for anything. We all laughed, happy over their ability to start to fight about trivial stuff because it meant that things were getting back to normal. They will be ok. Life is good! Health is great. And love is the best.

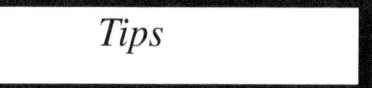

❖ To find out more about the S Factor, visit the website at sfactor.com and call your local gyms to find out if they offer the course.

❖ Learn more about the Lebed Method at Lebedmethod.com and Moving On Aerobics at movingonaerobics.org.

❖ A little preparation went a long way in getting me into the right attitude about starting up a new social life and dating.

I found it helpful to:

⇒ Practice what you will say to someone about your cancer story, anticipate how he or she might react and be ready with a response.

⇒ Think about dating as a learning process with the goal of having a social life you enjoy.

⇒ Not every date has to be perfect. If some people reject you (which can happen with or without cancer), you have not failed. Try to remember that not all dates worked out before you had cancer.

⇒ Remember, every woman deserves a man that calls her baby, kisses her like he means it, holds her tight like he never wants to let go, doesn't make her jealous with other women, instead makes other women jealous of her, is not afraid to let his friends know how he really feels about her and makes sure she knows how much he loves her.

⇒ Strength comes from confidence and experience, when you fall, pick yourself up and move on. Be determined. If a curve ball comes at you, hit it out of the damn park!

Chapter 8

STAY POSITIVE AND TAKE CONTROL: A FORMULA FOR HOPE

"I've learned that even when I have pains, I don't have to be one." — Maya Angelou

Laura Day's book, *Practical Intuition*, changed my life. It filled me with hope and taught me how to trust myself. Day suggests that regardless of the dilemma—work-related or personal—go with your gut. My gut gave me hope. It said that life is beautiful; it's a special gift and is definitely worth being lived. Day's book helped me reflect and decide what is truly important to me. I want a simple and happy life, shared with family and friends. I learned that I have the power to control my destiny and that I should have faith in my choices. If someone doesn't agree with those choices and moves on, I will have no regrets. Before cancer, I often put other people's issues first and put my own motivations and dreams on the back burner. Now I put 200 percent stock in rebuilding me from the inside out. This new focus has made me stronger. I beat cancer. I bought a home and rearranged my priorities to make myself truly happy.

We need to listen to our instincts and stay connected to the inner resources that can always move us in the right direction. Trusting my intuition helped me keep looking for the doctors and surgeons that were right for me. I controlled my destiny by seeking advice from cancer survivors and health professionals in order to get as much input as possible for making good decisions. I have met many people who have been cancer free for five or more years yet still dwell on their experiences in a negative way. They do not try to move on or reach out to others. They have not returned to work and blame cancer for making their lives miserable. I can't understand that attitude, and inside I shout to them, "You got a second chance! Take advantage of it!"

> *"Intuition should be an integral part of your life, like exercise or meditation. Employing it will open you up and add to the quality of both your thinking and your emotional selves."*
>
> *Excerpt From __Practical Intuition__ by Laura Day*

Having cancer inspired me to turn up the volume of my life. Moments go by very quickly and we don't get them back. As hard as the ordeal was, and as tough as it was to leave my comfort zone and break up with Michael in order to focus on my needs, the results are worth it. Cancer disrupted my life but at the same time it made me stronger. I saw how brave I could be. It made me appreciate every moment I have so much more. Only I can steer things the way I want them to go. I am accountable for everything I do and I love it that way.

I am Catholic and believe God exists. I believe in praying in your heart at all times, not just when you want something to happen. My last thought going to sleep and first thought waking up is to say thank God for this day. When I woke up from surgery I had lost my breasts, but I couldn't care less because I was so grateful to be alive.

Although it may be difficult to believe at the beginning, a breast cancer diagnosis can be empowering. There are some things you can control and others you cant. If you can take ownership of what you can control and make the most of what you do have you rather than

> *You don't drown by falling in water. You drown by staying there.*

what you don't. Then you can discover new aspects of yourself and clarify what you want out of life. That is what breast cancer did for me, and it has done the same for many other women. Emmy-winning actress Edie Falco, best known as Carmela Soprano on the HBO series "The Sopranos," is one of those. As a breast cancer survivor at age 40, she took action on a dream she had been holding on to for years. "Cancer has a way of making you re-prioritize," she said, referring to her decision to adopt a baby. Still single, she suddenly knew that it was time. "Every cell in my body needed and wanted to be a mother," she said. She adopted a baby boy in January 2005 and came to the conclusion that breast cancer was an important part of her life journey. Looking back at her decision to adopt, she realized, "Maybe this is the way my life is supposed to have turned out."

God gave me a great gift. Only after my bout with cancer did I learn to appreciate everything in life, from the simple pleasures of rain and the sunrise to great people who inspire me. I have become generous with others and with myself, which can appear to be two extremes: I enjoy helping people less fortunate and rewarding

> *"Obviously, it wasn't meant for me to die of cancer at 40. Every day my life surprises me, just like my cancer diagnosis surprised me. But roll with it. That's our job as humans."*
> *-Edie Falco, Actress*

myself with materialistic objects after an accomplishment, such as finishing each chemotherapy treatment. It feels good to give kids money when I hear the ice cream truck coming down the block and to help a couple with disabilities at a restaurant by paying their bill. My heart feels bigger than it ever has before, and that gives me hope for a future filled with love.

"The Obstacles In Our Path"

by Fern Field Brooks

In ancient times, a king had a boulder placed on a roadway. Then he hid himself and watched to see if anyone would remove the huge rock. Some of the king's wealthy merchants and courtiers came and simply walked around it. Many loudly blamed the king for not keeping the roads clear, but none did anything about getting the big stone out of the way.

Then a peasant came along carrying a load of vegetables. On approaching the boulder, the peasant laid down his burden and tried to move it. Pushing and straining he finally succeeded.

As the peasant picked up his load of vegetables he noticed a purse lying in the road where the boulder had been. The purse contained many gold coins and a note from the king indicating that the gold was for the person who removed the boulder from the roadway. The peasant learned what many people never understand:

Every obstacle presents an opportunity to improve one's condition.

Hope means many different things to me. It means my dreams coming true, such as having children one day. During and after cancer treatment, I chose to do everything my doctors told me to do so that I can stay strong and healthy and become a mother.

Positive Approaches

Instead of dwelling on the bad, I urge you to focus on all the good things in your life. I could choose to cry for days or I could clean out my closet and bring some clothes to the Goodwill store. I could stay in bed all day or call friends to come by and share a meal and stories. I could push all my fears and other uncomfortable feelings away or let them flow into a journal about my breast cancer experience. I could push all my cancer memories down and close that chapter or share everything I learned with other women to try to make their experiences easier.

According to scientific research, the act of writing about our breast cancer experience actually has a positive impact on our health. Studies have shown that writing down our thoughts, feelings and any benefits we perceive strengthens the immune

Remember:
You are brave and strong and you are someone's hero!

The Healing Power of a Breast Cancer Journal

It is a scientific fact that writing about our thoughts and feelings has a positive effect on our health.

Focusing on our selves in this way reduces stress and boosts the immune system. In a recent study, a group of women with breast cancer recorded, in 20-minute sessions, their deepest thoughts and feelings about their experience with breast cancer and any benefits they perceived from the experience. Another group of breast cancer patients—the control group—wrote about *non-personal, factual* aspects of breast cancer. At a three-month follow-up, the women who wrote about their thoughts, feelings and benefits had fewer physical symptoms than the control group.

Many other studies published over the past several years have shown that writing about valued aspects of the self, such as our thoughts and feelings, reduces stress and promotes health and well-being.

Take 15 or 20 minutes every day, or a few days a week, to describe your inner experience with breast cancer in a notebook or journal. As you quietly reflect on your self, know that your body is responding to this contemplation in a positive way by alleviating stress and strengthening your immune system. Researchers do not understand *why* self-reflection has this effect on the body, but they are certain that the effect is real.

Source: Personality and Social Psychology Bulletin, February 2007

system and lowers stress. Keeping a breast cancer journal, therefore, can be a powerful tool for healing.

Staying organized with all the paperwork involved in cancer treatment was another habit that helped me stay focused and positive. My good friend from work, Greta, who was a few months ahead of me in her cancer treatment, showed me the binder she had put together for herself and recommended that I make one. The binder, or the Book, contained sections for every aspect of my cancer care and experiences, and it was incredibly helpful.

Every time I got home from a doctor's appointment or trip to the drug store it was routine to put the receipts in the Book. This resource kept everything related to my medical condition in one place. By the time I had my first surgery the Book was so bulky and heavy that I left it at home.

I never had to search for a bill, phone number or co-pay receipt because every type of item had its place in the Book. This was empowering and I was proud of myself for being so organized and in control. Why make yourself crazy looking for a bill when you could be doing something that makes you feel good? When you have so

> *Our life is frittered away by detail. Simplify simplify, simplify!*
> *-Henry David Thoreau*

much on your plate, it's smart to simplify your life any way you can.

You will thank yourself time after time if you make your own Book as soon as possible. Pick up a three-inch binder, some tab divider pages, folders punched with three holes and a three-hole punch for papers that don't fit in the folders. Here is a description of the sections I created for my Book. Many of them may work for your own Book, but I invite you to tailor the list to the categories that fit your needs.

Organize and Simplify:
Suggested Sections for Your "Book"

BREAST SURGEON

Include a business card, CV (resume) and any other information you collect about this member of your medical team.

ONCOLOGIST

Same as above.

RECONSTRUCTIVE SURGEON

Same as above.

MASSAGE THERAPIST/ACCUPUNCTURIST

. . . or any other alternative health care practitioner. Keep a separate section for each caregiver and include the same documents you collected for members of your medical team.

INFORMATION

This section is for pamphlets and other materials about your condition and medical care. You may want to make separate sections for each topic. I printed out many pages from websites and filed them here for easy access.

CALENDAR

I preferred looking at an entire month at a time, but insert the type of calendar that suits you. You can print out free calendar pages from Yahoo and other websites. Keep track of your doctor appointments, chemotherapy sessions, meetings, dates for support groups, and anything else that comes up.

POST-CANCER CALENDAR

Make plans for activities that you will treat yourself to when you are finished with your treatments. This calendar constantly reminded me that I had a lot to look forward to and helped me keep an eye on my healthy future.

MEDICAL REPORTS

This includes materials that your doctors give you as well as notes you take during your appointments. I found that there was often so much information to take in during an appointment that I brought a tape recorder along and typed out the "report" later. Thorough, organized notes are very helpful when you discuss your condition and treatments with your family.

BILLS

There are several reasons to keep your bills handy and organized. Billing errors, like getting billed twice for the same service, can happen, and when you have all your documents you will be able to prove your case. You may also be eligible for tax credits for some of your medical bills, so you'll appreciate this section at tax time.

CO-PAYS

I created this section to keep tabs on how much my care was costing me out-of-pocket, and also to have a record in case of billing mistakes. Always get a receipt when you make a co-payment and store it here.

EXPENSES

This includes parking, taxi, toll and other transportation receipts and any other out-of-pocket expenses that come up during your treatment.

DISABILITY

I was fortunate to be able to file for disability at work and keep getting a paycheck while I wasn't working. If you are eligible for disability at work, this is where you can save copies of lab reports and other documents that you submit to your human resources department. It's a good backup in case the office loses something.

WELL WISHES

I loved turning to this section to look at all the cards and emails that I received during my cancer treatment. It never failed to cheer me up. I have shared Greta's idea for a resource book with many people. When the receptionist in one of my doctors' offices told me that her daughter-in-law had just been diagnosed with breast cancer, I told her about the Book and how much easier it made my life. She loved the idea and was grateful that I could pass along such useful information. When someone comes to me with a question about breast cancer, I am happy to have a wealth of information at my fingertips.

The Book became a good habit with me. I started up versions for home improvement, taxes and utilities, and the process has made me a little more organized in everything I do.

Getting organized is one way that my life has become more simple since I had cancer. Finding value in simplifying things reminds me of Henry David Thoreau's words in *Walden*: "I am convinced, both by faith and experience, that to maintain one's self on this earth is not a hardship but a pastime, if we will live simply and wisely." My new outlook is much like this because the gratitude in my heart makes life much lighter, like a pastime. I used to worry about the future, but now I live in the moment, because tomorrow may never come.

❖ A short list of recommended reading for exploring the connection between a positive attitude and healing:

> *Mind Over Malignancy: Living With Cancer* by Wayne D. Gersh, Ph.D., William L. Golden, Ph.D., and David M. Robbins, Ph.D.
>
> *Peace, Love and Healing: Bodymind Communication and the Path to Self-Healing* by Bernie Siegel, M.D.
>
> *Meditations for Enhancing Your Immune System: Strengthening Your Body's Ability to Heal* (audiobook) by Bernie Siegel.
>
> *The Cancer Conqueror: An Incredible Journey to Wellness* by Greg Anderson

❖ The entire article about the health benefits of writing about your breast cancer experience can be found at http://psp.sagepub.com/cgi/content/abstract/33/2/238 ("Does Self-Affirmation, Cognitive Processing, or Discovery of Meaning Explain Cancer-Related Health Benefits of Expressive Writing?" by J. David Creswell et al, *Personality and Social Psychology Bulletin,* Vol. 33 No. 2, February 2007, p. 238-250.)

ABOUT THE AUTHOR:

A native New Yorker, Judy San Roman has spent most of her adult career

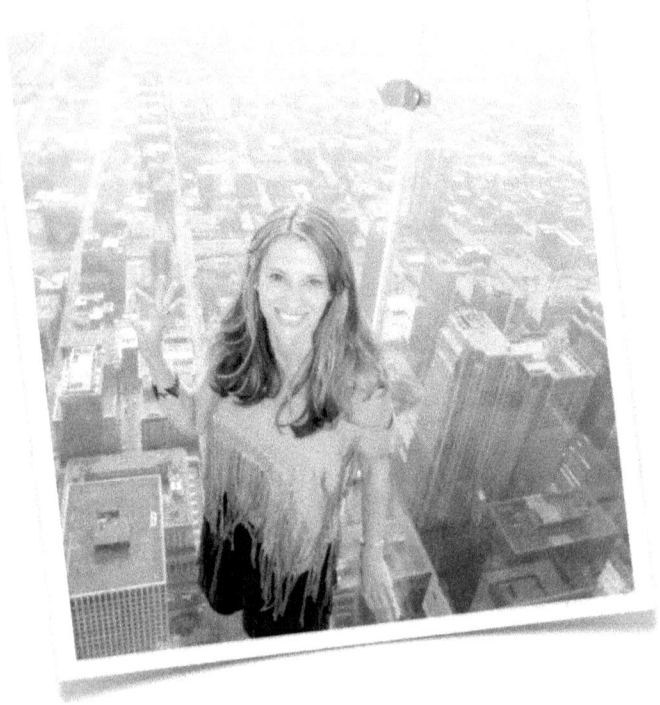

in pharmaceutical sales with one of America's biggest pharmaceutical companies. Since beating cancer in 2006, she has also been an inspirational speaker and advocate for women facing the same challenge. She is an avid writer of children's books and screenplays, and THEY'RE FAKE AND THEY'RE SPECTACULAR is her first nonfiction book.

Author's website: www.theyarefakeandtheyarespectacular.com

www.ingramcontent.com/pod-product-compliance
Lightning Source LLC
Chambersburg PA
CBHW071356310526
45789CB00020B/348